Trends in Wound Care
Volume V

Trends in Wound Care

Volume V

edited by

Keith F Cutting

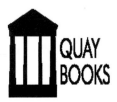

QUAY
BOOKS

Quay Books Division, MA Healthcare Ltd, St Jude's Church, Dulwich Road, London SE24 0PB

British Library Cataloguing-in-Publication Data
A catalogue record is available for this book

© MA Healthcare Limited 2009
ISBN 10: 1-85642-374-3
ISBN 13: 978-1-85642-374-8

Printed in the UK by CLE, St Ives, Huntingdon, Cambridgeshire

Contents

List of contributors   vi
Foreword   viii
Richard J White

1. A point prevalence survey of wounds in North East England   11
   N Srinivasaiah, H Dugdall, S Barrett and PJ Drew
2. A review of current objective and subjective scar assessment tools   27
   D Q A Nguyen, T Potokar and P Price
3. Evaluation of pH measurement as a method of wound assessment   39
   V K Shukla, D Shukla, S K Tiwary, S Agrawal and A Rastogi
4. The potential effect of fibroblast senescence on wound healing
   and the chronic wound environment   47
   E A Henderson
5. Nitric oxide restores impaired healing in normoglycaemic
   diabetic rats   57
   M Schäffer, M Bongartz, S Fischer, B Proksch and R Viebahn
6. An overview of the two widely accepted, but contradictory,
   theories on wound contraction   73
   S Pellard
7. A study of biofilm-based wound management in subjects
   with critical limb ischaemia   81
   R D Wolcott and D D Rhoads
8. Bacterial profiling using skin grafting, standard culture and
   molecular bacteriological methods   101
   A Andersen, KE Hill, P Stephens, DW Thomas,
   B Jorgensen and KA Krogfelt
9. The influence of essential oils on the process of wound healing:
   a review of the current evidence   115
   A C Woollard, K C Tatham and S Barker
10. Can translocated bacteria reduce wound infection?   125
    V I Nikitenko
11. Efficacy of TNP on lower limb wounds: A meta-analysis   133
    U Sadat, G Chang, A Noorani, S R Walsh, P D Hayes and K Varty

Index   143

List of contributors

S Agrawal, MBBS, Junior Resident, Department of Orthopaedics, Institute of Medical Sciences, Banaras Hindu University, Varanasi, India

A Andersen, MSc, Research Fellow, Department of Bacteriology, Mycology and Parasitology, ABMP, Statens Serum Institut, Copenhagen, Denmark and Copenhagen Wound Healing Centre, Bispebjerg University Hospital, Copenhagen, Denmark

S Barker, FRCS, Consultant Vascular Surgeon, University College London Hospital, London, UK

S Barrett, BSc (Hons), PGCM, RGN, Tissue Viability Nurse, East Riding of Yorkshire Primary Care Trust, UK

M Bongartz, PhD, Research Fellow, Department of Surgery, University Hospital of Tübingen, Germany

G Chang, MB BS, Surgical Intern, Cambridge Vascular Unit, Addenbrooke's Hospital, Cambridge University Hospitals NHS Foundation Trust, Cambridge, UK

K F Cutting, Principal Lecturer – Tissue Viability, Buckinghamshire New University, Buckinghamshire, UK

P J Drew, BSc, MD (Hons), MS, FRCS (Ed, Eng & Glas), FRCS (Gen), Professor/Honorary Consultant Surgeon, Hull York Medical School and Director of the Institute of Wound Care, University of Hull, UK

H Dugdall, BSc (Hons), MPhil, RGN, Practice Development Nurse, Tissue Viability, Hull and East Yorkshire Hospitals NHS Trust, UK

S Fischer, BS, Scientist, Department of Surgery, University Hospital of Tübingen, Germany

P D Hayes, MD, FRCS, Consultant Vascular Surgeon, Cambridge Vascular Unit, Addenbrooke's Hospital, Cambridge University Hospitals NHS Foundation Trust, Cambridge, UK

E A Henderson, BSc (Hons) Podiatry, PgD, Diabetes Specialist Podiatrist, Sunderland Royal Hospital, Sunderland, UK

K E Hill, PhD, Senior Research Fellow, Wound Biology Group, Cardiff Institute of Tissue Engineering and Repair, Oral Surgery, Medicine and Pathology, Cardiff University, UK

B Jorgensen, MD, Senior Registrar, Copenhagen Wound Healing Centre, Bispebjerg University Hospital, Copenhagen, Denmark

K A Krogfelt, PhD, Professor of Medical Microbiology, Department of Bacteriology, Mycology and Parasitology, ABMP, Statens Serum Institut, Copenhagen, Denmark

D Q A Nguyen, MB, ChB, MRCS (Eng), Specialist Registrar in Burns and
Plastic Surgery, Department of Burns and Plastic Surgery, Morriston
Hospital, Swansea, Wales, UK

V I Nikitenko, DM, Professor, Department of Trauma Surgery, Orthopaedics
and Military Surgery, Orenburg State Medical Academy, Russia

A Noorani, MRCS, Senior House Officer, Cambridge Vascular Unit,
Addenbrooke's Hospital, Cambridge University Hospitals NHS Foundation
Trust, Cambridge, UK

S Pellard, BSc, MB Ch, MRCS (Eng), GP Registrar, Cardiff, UK

T Potokar, FRCS (plast), Consultant Burns and Reconstructive Surgeon,
Department of Burns and Plastic Surgery, Morriston Hospital, Swansea,
Wales, UK

P Price, BA (Hons), PhD, AFBPsS, CHPsychol, Director of Academic
Research and Education, Wound Healing Unit and Non-clinical Professor,
Cardiff University, Wales, UK

B Proksch, BS, Scientist, Department of Surgery, University Hospital,
Knappschaftskrankenhaus Bochum-Langendreer, Germany

A Rastogi, MS, Reader, Department of Orthopaedics, Institute of Medical
Sciences, Banaras Hindu University, Varanasi, India

D D Rhoads, MT(ASCP)CM, Laboratory Research Coordinator, Southwest
Regional Wound Care Center, Lubbock, Texas US

U Sadat, MRCS, Fellow in Vascular Surgery, Cambridge Vascular Unit,
Addenbrooke's Hospital, Cambridge University Hospitals NHS Foundation
Trust, Cambridge, UK

M Schäffer, MD, Consultant Surgeon, Department of Surgery, University
Hospital, Knappschaftskrankenhaus Bochum-Langendreer, Germany

D Shukla, MBBS, Junior Resident, Department of General Surgery, Institute of
Medical Sciences, Banaras Hindu University, Varanasi, India

V K Shukla, MS, Mch (Wales), Professor and Head, Department of General
Surgery, Institute of Medical Sciences, Banaras Hindu University, Varanasi,
India

N Srinivasaiah, MRCS (Eng, Ed, Glas), MRCSI (Dub), (DNB-Ind), Research
Fellow, Academic Surgical Unit, Castle Hill Hospital, University of Hull,
UK

P Stephens PhD, Reader in Cell Biology, Wound Biology Group, Cardiff
Institute of Tissue Engineering and Repair, Oral Surgery, Medicine and
Pathology, Cardiff University, UK

K C Tatham, BSc (Hons), MBBS, Anaesthetic Senior House Officer, Ealing

Hospital NHS Trust, London, UK

D W Thomas, MD, PhD, Professor of Oral Surgery, Wound Biology Group, Cardiff Institute of Tissue Engineering and Repair, Oral Surgery, Medicine and Pathology, Cardiff University, UK

S K Tiwary, MS, Senior Resident, Department of General Surgery, Institute of Medical Sciences, Banaras Hindu University, Varanasi, India

K Varty, MD, FRCS, Consultant Vascular Surgeon, Cambridge Vascular Unit, Addenbrooke's Hospital, Cambridge University Hospitals NHS Foundation Trust, Cambridge, UK

R Viebahn, MD, Clinical Director Surgeon, Department of Surgery, University Hospital, Knappschaftskrankenhaus Bochum-Langendreer, Germany

S R Walsh, MRCS, Specialist Registrar, Cambridge Vascular Unit, Addenbrooke's Hospital, Cambridge University Hospitals NHS Foundation Trust, Cambridge, UK

R D Wolcott, MD, CWS, Director, Southwest Regional Wound Care Center, Lubbock, Texas US

A C Woollard, BSc (Hons), BM, MRCS, Plastics Senior House Officer, St George's Hospital, London, UK

Foreword

It is testimony to the growing interest in wound management that the *Trends* series has reached Volume V in barely as many years. This highly reputable source of up-to-date monographs has become a standard text for those seeking to keep in touch with key areas of clinical and scientific research. The current volume, edited by Keith Cutting, maintains the established standard. It contains an eclectic miscellany of chapters, each based upon published (and so, peer-reviewed) articles from journals in the MA Healthcare collection. Where important new information has been published, chapters have been updated accordingly; thus, this volume is of 2009 vintage.

The editor has included something for those with a practical focus as well as new science and theoretical debate. Such disparate topics as wound survey/audit, topical negative pressure, bacterial profiling and biofilms, wound pH, scar assessment, fibroblast senescence, the role of nitric oxide, and theories on wound contraction are covered.

For example, the growing interest in topical negative pressure is reflected by the inclusion of a meta-analysis updated to incorporate the most recent data available. This chapter is an excellent baseline for all wishing to update their knowledge on clinical evidence in this exciting field. Chapters on wound microbiology and biofilms similarly reflect what is, in my opinion, the most fascinating area of chronic wound pathophysiology. These chapters illustrate just how far our understanding has come in the past decade, and just how important it is for clinicians to be aware of the latest developments in wound microbiology and infection if they are to provide 'best practice' care.

This collection of chapters shows how our chosen field has progressed in recent years, and, helps busy clinicians keep appraised of important research.

Richard White
Professor of Tissue Viability
Institute of Health and Society
University of Worcester, UK.

CHAPTER 1

A point prevalence survey of wounds in North East England

N Srinivasaiah, H Dugdall, S Barrett and P J Drew

Wounds represent a major burden in terms of morbidity and reduced quality of life for patients and their carers, and a drain on health-care resources (Cully, 1008). They are a significant problem in both hospital and domestic settings, affecting people of all ages, social class and race. Pain, discomfort, low self-esteem and poor body image can cause personal suffering (Cully, 1998). Osteomyelitis and life-threatening sepsis are associated major complications (Cully, 1998).

Several guidelines have been published to promote better wound management practice. They include the Royal College of Nursing's clinical guidelines on pressure ulcer prevention and the management of venous leg ulcers (Royal College of Nursing, 2008), the National Institute of Health and Clinical Excellence guidelines on debriding agents, diabetic foot care and pressure ulcer care (National Institute for Health and Clinical Excellence, 2001a, b, 2004), and the Scottish Intercollegiate Guidelines Network (SIGN) (2008) recommendations on the management of diabetic foot disease and the care of patients with chronic leg ulcers.

It is an essential requirement to have a baseline measurement of wound care in order to monitor practice and ascertain if national and regional guidelines are in place and being adhered to. In May 2005, the wound-care audit team in Hull and East Yorkshire, located in the north-east region of the UK, conducted a point prevalence audit which aimed to:

- Review current wound-care practice and the standard of wound care.
- Obtain information on prevalence, treatment and outcomes.
- Provide a basis for estimating the extent of the problem, treatment modalities used, service provision and future needs.
- Highlight areas of care in need of improvement.
- Highlight areas with excellent wound practices.
- Gain valuable information for future research projects.

This chapter describes the audit, its findings and recommendations for improvements.

Method

A team of tissue viability nurses (TVNs) and audit staff within the catchment area conducted the prevalence audit. The five trusts covered by the audit were: West Hull Primary Care Trust (PCT) and Eastern Hull PCT (now combined to form Hull PCT), Yorkshire Wolds and Coast PCT, East Yorkshire PCT (now combined to form East Riding of Yorkshire PCT), and Hull and East Yorkshire Hospitals NHS Trust. The trusts have a combined population of approximately 590 000.

The audit forms

There were two types of data-collection forms. First, one which gathered information on total bed occupancy or the number of patients registered at each district nurse base on the day of the audit. Second, a specific wound-care audit form which was completed for each patient with a wound.

Data were gathered on the professional treating the wound, the geographical location in which treatment was provided, patient comorbidities, number of wounds on each patient, the wound type, wound assessment, suspected wound infection and reasons for undertaking a swab. Information was gathered on the reference wound including exudate levels, wound bed characteristics, pressure ulcer prevention strategies used, pressure-redistributing equipment, dressings used and patient concordance.

The audit forms were developed by the local wound-care experts and were based on clinical experience. Data were gathered from the patients' notes and via verbal feedback from key staff caring for the patients. Wounds were not inspected for the purposes of the audit.

If a patient had more than one wound, data were collected only on the most serious wound (the 'reference' wound), as judged by the clinician caring for the patient.

A small pilot study was undertaken to ensure the forms were acceptable in terms of ease of use. In addition, TVNs were questioned on the same patient sample to determine whether the responses were consistent in relation to appropriate, inappropriate or unsafe dressing usage. Following the pilot it was agreed that the data collection tool was fit for purpose without any alterations.

Data collection

Data were collected from the region's acute trust and its primary care trusts, nursing and residential homes, hospice and local prisons.

In the acute hospital trust, a TVN and a member of the audit department visited each ward over a two-day period to gather data from ward nurses on all inpatients with a wound. A TVN also collected data in this way from the local hospice.

On the same date, all district nurses employed by the PCTs were asked to provide data on every patient with a wound on their active caseload.

Meanwhile, senior staff from the nursing homes, the local hospice and Hull and East Riding prisons collected data on all of their patients with wounds, which were then reported to a visiting TVN.

Data entry and analysis

The audit was coordinated by the clinical effectiveness department of West Hull PCT and the clinical audit department of Hull and East Yorkshire Hospitals NHS Trust. Data analysis was performed using SPSS software. Descriptive analysis and cross tabulations were also used. The clinical governance department ensured the full audit process was conducted to an acceptable standard.

Results

Response rates

A total of 1645 forms, relating to 1644 wounds, were received: 1291 from the primary care trusts (PCTs), prisons and nursing and residential homes (16 of the 32 nursing and residential homes responded), and 354 from the acute trust and hospice.

As stated above, the intention was to include data on the reference wound only. However, some participants returned more than one form per patient, which is reflected in the prevalence figures given below. This is discussed in more detail in the study limitations section in the discussion.

Wound prevalence

The cumulative wound prevalence for the region was 12%. Prevalence rates for the different settings are given in *Figure 1*. The acute trust had a prevalence rate of 27%, while the PCT rates ranged from 7% to 17%. Prevalence in the nursing and residential homes was 12%, while prisons had the lowest rate of 1%.

Wound type

Surgical wounds were the most common type (n=699, 41.5%), followed by leg and foot ulcers (n=629, 37.3%) and then pressure ulcers (n=294, 17.4%). Full details are given in *Table 1*. Most of the surgical wounds (31.4%) were primary closures.

Wound duration

Most of the 1644 wounds (44.1%) were six weeks old or less; 14.8% were at least one year old, including 28% of the leg and foot ulcers, but only 7% of the surgical wounds.

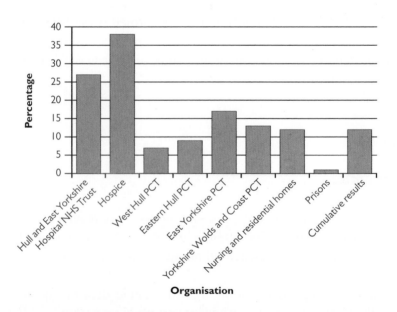

Figure 1. Percentage of patients with wounds in different settings within Hull and East Yorkshire.

Table 1. Number and percentage of wounds per patient by wound type

	Wound type					
	Leg and foot ulcers		Pressure ulcers		Surgical wounds	
	Number	(%)	Number	(%)	Number	(%)
1 wound/person	400	(63.6)	181	(61.9)	525	(75)
2 wounds/person	141	(22.4)	70	(23.8)	117	(16.7)
3 wounds/person	44	(7.0)	25	(8.5)	30	(4.3)
4 wounds/person	13	(2.1)	10	(3.4)	9	(1.3)
5 wounds/person	8	(1.3)	2	(0.7)	3	(0.4)
6 wounds/person	2	(0.3)	2	(0.7)	3	(0.4)
Other	13	(2.1)	2	(0.7)	6	(0.9)
Healed	3	(0.5)	0	(0.0)	0	(0.0)
NDS	5	(0.8)	1	(0.3)	6	(0.9)
Total	629	(100)	294	(100)	699	(100)

Other = seven or more wounds
NDS = no data supplied

Wound infections

A total of 211 (12.8%) of the 1644 wounds were considered to be clinically infected. Some 1367 (83.2%) had no infection, 16 (1%) 'didn't know whether the wound was infected or not', 19 (1.2%) did not undergo wound assessment, and 31 (1.9%) had no data supplied. Of the 211 wounds considered infected, the most common clinical signs of infections (48–50.2%) described by the respondents were pus, erythema and malodour. Other clinical signs cited included wound pallor and fever. In all, 128 of the 211 wounds (60.7%) had been swabbed for culture. Fifty-three of the wounds not considered infected (3.9%) also had a swab sent for culture.

Pressure ulcers

There were 294 pressure ulcers, of which 12.6% were classified as grade 1, 37.4% as grade 2, 19.7% as grade 3 and 4.1% grade 4. Of the rest, 1.5% were classified as eschar and 24.7% did not have grade data supplied.

Risk categories and equipment

Different risk assessment tools were used in the acute trust and in the community. Waterlow score (Bridel, 1993) was used in the acute trust and a mixture of Waterlow and Walsall scores (Milward et al., 1993) were used in the community.

Equipment

Of 294 patients with pressure ulcers, just over half (56%) received some form of pressure-redistributing mattress. Twelve of the 16 patients (75%) with a grade 4 pressure ulcer used a powered pressure-redistributing mattress.

Repositioning schedule

Of the 294 patients with a pressure ulcer, 149 (51%) had a repositioning schedule. This varied with grade, with 47% of patients with grade 1 and 2 ulcers, 59% of those with grades 3 and 4, and 75% with a grade 4 ulcer having repositioning schedules.

Table 2. Wound characteristics

Wound type	Number	(%)
Leg and foot ulcers		
Venous ulcer	260	37.6
Arterial ulcer	86	12.4
Mixed (venous/arterial)	86	12.4
Neuropathic	43	4.9
Do not know	78	11.3
Other	85	12.3
NDS	63	9.1
Total	692	100
Surgical wounds		
Primary closure	239	31.4
Open	136	17.8
Dehisence	74	9.7
Trauma wound	191	25.1
Other	59	7.7
NDS	63	16.2
Total	762	100

NDS = no data supplied

Risk assessment scores/bed and chairs

A total of 51.6% (n=115) of the static and dynamic pressure-redistributing mattresses used were allocated to 'very high risk' (Waterlow) or 'high risk' (Walsall) patients. A further 24.7% (n=55) were allocated to patients in the next risk category, 'high risk' (Waterlow) or 'medium risk' (Walsall). The remaining 23.7% (n=53) were allocated to patients classed 'not at risk' and 'low risk' (Walsall) and 'at risk' (Waterlow).

Leg and foot ulcers

Of the 629 leg or foot ulcers, 163 (25.9%) had no definitive diagnosis of the underlying aetiology. Leg ulcer aetiologies are given in *Table 2*. (The discrepancies between *Tables 1* and *Table 2* are due to the fact that some respondents returned data on more than one wound.)

Use of Doppler

Of the 692 leg and foot wounds, the aetiology was recorded in 466 cases. Most were classified as venous (37.6%), followed by arterial (12.4%) and mixed aetiology (12.4%).

Of the 466 ulcers with a recorded aetiology, 129 (27.7%) had not been assessed using Doppler. Just over three-quarters (78.8%) of the 260 venous leg ulcers were assessed with Doppler, compared with 20.6% of the neuropathic ulcers (Table 3). Doppler was used on just over half (51.5%) of the 692 leg and foot ulcers.

Diabetes

In all, 29.6% of the patients with a foot ulcer had diabetes. Of the 162 wounds on the foot or heel, the diabetes status was known in only 105 (64.8%). A total of 115 of patients (18.3%) with a leg or foot ulcer were recorded as having diabetes.

Compression

Of the 260 reported venous leg ulcers, 208 (80%) received compression, of which 139 (66.8%) were given multilayer high compression. Thirty (34.9%) of the patients with mixed aetiology ulcers were given compression (*Table 3*).

Dressings

Most of primary and secondary dressings used were non-adherent or low-adherent contact wound dressings at 25.9% and 27.3% respectively.

Table 3. Use of Doppler and compression

	Total	Assessed using Doppler?		Compression used?				
		Yes	No	Yes	No	Refused	NDS	N/A
		No. (%)	No. (%)	No. (%)	No. (%)	No. (%)	No. (%)	No. (%)
Venous ulcer	260	205 (78.8)	55 (21.2)	208 (80)	32 (12)	0 (0)	20 (7.7)	0 (0)
Arterial ulcer	86	58 (67.4)	28 (32.6)	6 (7)	72 (84)	1 (1.2)	7 (8.1)	0 (0)
Mixed aetiology	86	67 (77.9)	19 (21.1)	30 (34.9)	53 (61.6)	0 (0)	3 (3.5)	0 (0)
Neuropathic	34	7 (20.6)	27 (79.4)	0 (0)	31 (91.2)	0 (0)	3 (8.8)	0 (0)
Don't know	78	4 (5.1)	74 (94.9)	8 (10.3)	59 (75.6)	0 (0)	11 (14.1)	0 (0)
NDS	63	4 (6.3)	59 (93.7)	5 (7.9)	29 (46)	0 (0)	29 (46)	0 (0)
Other type of leg and foot ulcers	85	9 (10.6)	76 (89.4)	6 (7.1)	73 (85.9)	0 (0)	6 (7.1)	0 (0)
Other wounds (pressure ulcers and surgical wounds)	952	20 (2.1)	932 (97.9)	21 (2.2)	685 (72)	0 (0)	244 (25.6)	2 (2)
Total	1644	374 (22.7)	1270 (77.3)	284 (17.3)	1034 (62.9)	1 (1)	323 (19.6)	2 (1)

Primary dressings and exudate levels

The main findings on appropriateness of dressings used related to exudate levels and are summarised below.

Exudate levels
Of the 1644 wounds, 344 (21%) had no exudate, 703 (42.8%) had low levels of exudate, 399 (24.2%) had medium levels and 101 (6.1%) had high levels. The remaining wounds were either not assessed or no data were supplied. Exudate levels were determined by the clinician into categories of high, medium, low and none.

Acceptable practice
Of the 344 wounds with no exudate, 111 (32.3%) were dressed with a non- or low-adherent dressing and 36 (10.5%) a film dressing.

Concerns within practice
Of the 703 patients with low exudate levels, 128 (18.2%) were given an antimicrobial/iodine dressing. Meanwhile, six of the 101 patients (5.9%) with high exudate levels were given a hydrogel dressing.

Primary dressings and the appearance of the wound bed

A summary of the results is presented below.

Appearance of the wound bed
Of the 1644 wounds, most were granulating (61.4%), followed by epithelialising (28%), sloughy (32.7%), necrotic (4.4%) and fungating (0.8%). Most wounds (41.9%) were located on the lower leg. *Figure 2* shows the top seven locations of the reference wound.

Acceptable practice
Twenty of the 73 necrotic wounds (27.4%) and 100 of the 539 sloughy wounds (18.6%) were given hydrogel dressings. Eighty-four (15.6%) of the sloughy wounds had a silver-impregnated Hydrofiber dressing.
 Of the 1010 granulating wounds, 260 (25.7%) were given a non-adherent or low-adherent contact wound dressing.

Concerns within practice
Of the 1010 patients with a granulating wound, 142 (14.1%) were given an

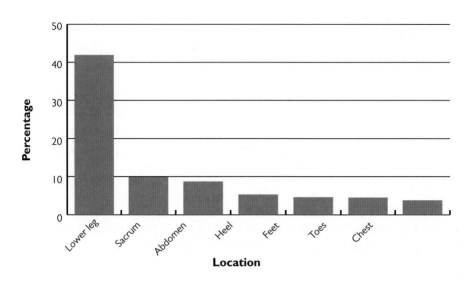

Figure 2. Position on the body of the most serious wounds.

antimicrobial/iodine dressing, as were 67 of the 463 patients (14.5%) with an epithelialising wound. Twenty-eight patients (2.8%) with a granulating wound were given an alginate dressing.

Cleansing

Just over two-thirds (68%) of the wounds were cleansed, with saline being the most frequently used cleansing agent.

Professionals

Some 70.1% of the community nurses' workload involved wound care, with just over half (52.7%) of these wounds being treated in the patient's home. In the acute trust, surgical wounds were most commonly reported (62%).

Comorbidities

Of the 1644 patients with wounds, 15.1% had diabetes, 9.7% had a carcinoma; 16.1% had one or more of the following diseases: diabetes, vascular disease, rheumatoid disease, carcinoma or a neurological deficit.

Patient concordance and assessment

Most patients consented to treatment, with only 3.6% declining.

Within the hospital trust only 1.2% of wounds had not been assessed at the time of the audit. Visual observations, nursing history and physical examinations were the three most common methods of diagnosis used. Others included medical history, Doppler examination and biopsy.

Discussion

This audit gives an insight into the nature of wound care in the community and hospital, and an opportunity to identify areas in need of improvement.

Prevalence

Before this study, no equivalent study has been performed on such a large scale, covering both acute and community trusts, to determine a baseline prevalence of wound care in such a large geographic area. However, a prevalence study conducted in the community in the UK estimated the point prevalence of leg and foot ulcers to be in the region of 1.48/1000 population (Callam et al., 1985). The global prevalence of 'sores' was 8.3%, while that of pressure ulcers was 6.4% and leg ulcers 1.6%. In a prevalence study of primary care, rehabilitation units and long-term care units in a region in France, Caron-Mazet et al. (2007) quoted a global prevalence of 'chronic wounds' of 8.3%, while that of pressure ulcers was 6.4% and leg ulcers 1.6%.

Our results highlight several areas of concern. Almost half the patients with venous leg ulcers (46%) did not receive multilayer bandage systems; of those who did, 67% used multilayer high compression systems. Seven per cent of those with an arterial ulcer received compression. Diabetes status was not known in just over one-third (35%).

In addition, 3.9% of patients without clinical signs of infection were swabbed. Unnecessary swabs have a significant impact on already stretched resources: the local cost for providing a single swab result is approximately £18.

Wound care is a multidisciplinary practice, where prescriptions are generated by both nurses and doctors. However, nurses are predominantly responsible for the application of wound dressings. This audit identified areas of weakness related to wound assessment and consequently inappropriate dressing selection. For example, some highly exuding wounds were treated with a hydrogel, while granulating and epithelialising wounds were given antimicrobial/iodine dressings. There were also reports of alginates being used on granulating wounds. Various studies have shown that nurses and doctors working in the community need to update their knowledge of wound treatments (Haram et al., 2003a). Studies also indicate that nurses rely on experience and colleagues as the main sources of knowledge (Haram et al., 2003b).

The results of this audit suggest that effective and timely diagnosis and appropriate treatment could have a significant impact on wound care.

However, there were examples of good clinical practice. Most wounds were given the appropriate dressing for their level of exudate and tissue type. Non-exuding wounds were treated primarily with non- or low-adherent dressings, followed by film dressings. Similarly, most necrotic and sloughy wounds were treated with hydrogels, followed by a silver-impregnated hydrocolloid dressing in sloughy wounds, while most granulating wounds were given a non-adherent contact wound dressing.

Good response rates were achieved, mainly because the TVNs targeted the team leaders and collected the forms in person. A 100% response rate was achieved from the acute hospital, where the TVNs collected the audit forms directly from staff on the wards. As the TVNs did not inspect the wounds, relying instead on nursing documentation, there are instances where potentially inappropriate dressing selection could not be verified.

Clinical recommendations

Tissue viability services need to be supported by adequate resources in order to deliver educational packages that meet the needs of nursing and medical practitioners. This would also enhance service provision and patient care. This involves identifying and acting on organisational and clinical factors that influence delivery of best practice, as illustrated in Lorimer et al.'s (2003) study on venous leg ulcer care.

Develop a standardised, evidence-based, wound assessment tool for use in both primary and secondary care. The East Riding of Yorkshire PCT has since adopted and adapted the applied wound management tool (Wounds UK, 2008) to improve the quality of wound assessment to allow the practitioner to assess, plan, treat and document their actions. It standardises wound assessment across the PCTs, and introduced the Heal

---

Box 1. Suggestions for audit improvement

- Collect more detail on wound swabbing, such as routine screening, MRSA screening, pre-operative screening, immunosuppressed patients
- Collect data on primary reason for admission
- Collect data on delayed discharge if wound related
- Include the location where wounds developed – in particular, whether patients developed their wound in the present care setting or elsewhere
- Improve monitoring of response rates by recording which individuals did and did not respond
- Include/encourage involvement from GP practices
- Complete more accurately data-collection forms by maintaining uniformity in data collection by using one method across the community and acute trusts
- Address impact of wounds on quality of life, emphasising the patient's perspective and psychological aspects using a validated health-related quality-of-life (HRQoL) questionnaire.

Not Hurt tool from Mölnlycke Health Care to improve and standardise management of wound pain. Other participating trusts are considering implementation of these tools.

Reduce use of inappropriate wound-care products via evidence-based education, increasing awareness and focusing on practical skills relating to wound assessment and dressing application

Doppler assessment and diagnosis of arterial flow in leg ulcers needs to be addressed.

Limitations

Some data-quality issues occurred. In 41 forms it was identified that two or more wounds were significant. This was due to misinterpretation of the question in the audit tool by the practitioner. The local wound-care experts did not inspect the wounds due to time constraints and lack of resources. Suspected wound infections were not confirmed by swab results. GP practice nurses declined to take part in the study due to lack of resources.

Attempts will be made in future to overcome these limitations and to improve wound care. Suggestions for improving the audit process are listed in *Box 1*.

Conclusion

This point prevalence wound-care audit has helped the Institute of Wound Care to identify the prevalence, treatment practices and outcomes of current wound diagnosis and dressing provisions. It shows that such an audit can be successfully performed, while the data should be generalisable.

The audit has highlighted the need for effective and timely diagnosis and appropriate treatment, as well as the importance of evidence-based education, service provision and defined protocols and guidelines to improve the management structure for treating patients with wounds.

References

Bridel J (1003) Assessing the risk of pressure sores. *Nurs Stand* **7**: 32–5

Callam M, Ruckley CV, Harper DR, Dale JJ (1985) Chronic ulceration of the leg: Extent of the problem and provision of care. *Br Med J (Clin Res Ed)* **290**: 1855–6

Caron-Mazet J, Roth B, Guillaume JC (2007) Prevalence and management of chronic wounds in 14 geriatric institutions of the Haut-Rhin. *Ann Dermatol Venereol* **134**: 645–51

Culley F (1998) Nursing aspects of pressure sore prevention and therapy. *Br J Nurs* **7**: 879–86

Dale JJ, Callam MJ, Ruckley CV et al. (1983) Chronic ulcers of the leg: A study of prevalence in a Scottish community. *Health Bull (Edinb)* **41**: 310–14

Haram RB, Ribu E, Rustoen T (2003a) An evaluation of the leg and foot ulcer treatment provided in Oslo. *J Wound Care* **12**: 290–4

Haram R, Ribu E, Rustoen T (2003b) The views of district nurses on their level of knowledge about the treatment of leg and foot ulcers. *J Wound Ostomy Continence Nurs* **30**: 25–32

Lorimer KR, Harrison MB, Graham ID et al. (2003) Venous leg ulcer care: How evidence-based is nursing practice? *J Wound Ostomy Continence Nurs* **30**: 132–42

Milward P, Poole M, Skitt T (1993) Pressure sore prevention: Scoring pressure sore risk in the community. *Nurs Stand* **8**: 50–5

National Institute for Health and Clinical Excellence (2001a) *Wound care - debriding agents* (Technology appraisal). Available from: http://guidance.nice.org.uk/TA24

National Institute for Health and Clinical Excellence (2001b) *Pressure ulcers: pressure ulcer risk assessment and prevention* (clinical guideline). Available from: http://guidance.nice.org.uk/CGB

National Institute for Health and Clinical Excellence (2004) *Type 2 diabetes - footcare* (clinical guideline). Available from: http://guidance.nice.org.uk/CG10

Nelzen O, Bergqvist D, Lindhagen A, Hallbook T (1991) Chronic leg ulcers: An underestimated problem in primary health care among elderly patients. *J Epidemiol Community Health* **45**: 184–7

Royal College of Nursing (2008) *Clinical guidelines: venous leg ulcers*. Available from: www.rcn. org.uk/resources/guidelines.php [Accessed 10 July 2008]

Scottish Intercollegiate Guidelines Network (SIGN) (2008) Available from: www.sign.ac.uk/ guidelines/published/index.html [Accessed 10 July 2008]

Wounds UK (2008) *Applied Wound Management*. Available from: http://www.wounds-uk.com/ applied_wound_management.shtml. [Accessed 10 July 2008]

CHAPTER 2

A review of current objective and subjective scar assessment tools

D Q A Nguyen, T Potokar and P Price

Skin functions as a shield from the outside world, protecting our body from microorganisms, fluid loss and mechanical forces such as traction and shear. It plays a vital role in thermoregulation and its appearance is integral to our everyday social interactions. In the past, wound healing aimed to achieve rapid closure, whereas now the quality of the product of wound healing is becoming increasingly important, with more emphasis on functional and cosmetic outcomes.

A scar is the sum of the injury, the reparative process and subsequent interventions to improve the scarring process (Powers et al., 1999). It may have long lasting functional, cosmetic and psychological consequences for the patient. Scars have both objective — and thereby potentially quantitative — and subjective aspects.

Objective aspects include its physical characteristics, such as size, shape, area, volume, colour, texture and pliability.

Subjective aspects include various factors that contribute to the person's own evaluation of the scar, including their emotional reaction to the injury, changes in body image and social support.

Irrespective of the actual nature of the scar and the functional limitations that may affect it, the patient's perception of the scar can influence both quality of life and the clinical outcome (Powers et al., 1999).

An ideal scar assessment should try to include both the objective and subjective aspects of the scar. When evaluating any tool, it is important to consider biometric properties such as its reliability, sensitivity and validity. Reliability refers to the reproducibility of measurements or ratings by observers, as well as the accuracy of the tool (Streiner and Norman, 1989).

To evaluate various scar treatments, an assessment tool must also be sensitive enough to capture the changes in the scar and its effects over time (Powers et al., 1999). The ideal assessment tool should be:

- Easy to perform
- Painless
- Non-invasive
- Inexpensive.

This literature review aims to evaluate currently available scar assessment tools, with a view to establishing empirical evidence for wound healing and scar management therapies. The OVID and PubMed database, which includes Medline, Embase and Cinahl, was searched (from 1966 to 2000) using the following key words: scar assessment; scar evaluation; burn scar assessment; burn scar evaluation; scar measurement; Vancouver scar scale.

Subjective scar assessment

Subjective scar assessment scales have been developed to give an overall impression of the quality of the scar. The one most commonly used for burn scars is the Vancouver scar scale (VSS) (*Table 1*). This was the first attempt to standardise scar assessment (Sullivan et al., 1990). The scale scored pigmentation, vascularity, pliability and scar height, with the sum of the scores resulting in a number, which was bigger for hypertrophic scars. The VSS was subsequently modified to assess mixed pigmentation, pain and itching (Baryza and Baryza, 1995; Yeong et al., 1997).

Although the VSS is the most widely accepted and evaluated burn scar assessment scale, its reliability and validity have been questioned (Van Zuijlen et al., 2001). The original authors reported that its overall interrater reliability was good (Cohen's kappa coefficient [k] of 0.5) (Sullivan et al., 1990), but others have considered it to be moderate (Brennan and Silman, 1992).

The validity of the VSS is questionable as it is unclear why all the parameters have a maximum score of 3, apart from pliability, which has a maximum score of 5. Although pliability is an important functional aspect of a scar, there is no evidence this is more significant than other features such as pain, scar height, pigmentation or vascularity.

The VSS rating of pigmentation also has limitations. The assignment of a higher score for hyperpigmentation than hypopigmentation, and the implication that it is associated with an inferior overall outcome has been challenged (Nedelec et al., 2000). Oliveira et al. (2005) observed highly variable patterns of pigmentation in a significant percentage of hypertrophic and non-hypertrophic scars, and so did not include it in their rating scale.

Table 1. Vancouver scar scale

Vascularity	Normal = 0
	Pink = 1
	Red = 2
	Purple = 3
Pigmentation	Normal = 0
	Hypopigmentation = 1
	Mixed = 2
	Hyperpigmentation = 3
Pliability	Normal = 0
	Supple = 1
	Yielding = 2
	Firm = 3
	Ropes = 4
Height	Flat = 0
	<2mm = 1
	2–5mm = 2
	>5mm = 3

Although easy to use, the clinical utility of the VSS can be limited because it requires two or more observers to obtain meaningful data (Van Zuijlen et al., 2002).

Finally, the VSS provides ordinal data and hence it is not truly a scale.

Scar rating tools generally rate the scar from the perspective of the practitioner, not the patient. Martin et al. (2003) explored the relationship between the patients' and therapists' evaluations scarring. Twenty consecutive patients were recruited early after a burn injury and asked to rate their scars on a visual analogue scale (VAS) and to state their perception of how other people viewed it. A burn scar therapist, who was blinded to the VAS scores, concurrently performed a VSS assessment. This process was repeated 18 months later.

The findings showed that the VSS measurement bore no relationship to the patients' initial opinion of their scar. However, after 18 months the patients' feelings about their scars appeared to improve and correlate better with the VSS, although their impression of what other people thought about the scare still bore no relationship to the VSS rating. This suggests that patients were still unable to completely accept their scars, despite an objective improvement in scar quality (Martin et al, 2003).

This highlights the importance of taking the patient's perception of their scar into account during assessment, and it cannot be assumed that a 'good' scar is also viewed favourably by the patient. However, the finding that there was an improvement over time in the correlation between patients' opinions about their scars and VSS scores should be viewed with caution as only eight out of 20 patients were available for re-revaluation (four were lost to follow-up and eight declined to attend). This is a significant confounding factor (Crombie, 1996).

A study on breast cancer surgery scars (n=59) demonstrated that patient satisfaction was not associated with the VSS score but instead with self-ratings of scar pliability and pain. The authors concluded that it is important not only to evaluate patients' symptoms, but also their opinions about and overall satisfaction with their scar during assessment (Truong et al., 2005). However, the inclusion of multiple scars on multiple sites (breast and axilla) in the study may have introduced an element of bias as it may be difficult for patients to evaluate these independently of each other. In addition, the use of 12 observers may have had a detrimental effect on the reliability of the VSS scores and thus of the study findings.

The patient and observer scar assessment scale incorporates the patient's perspective of their scar, making it more suitable for clinical scar evaluation studies (Draaijers et al., 2004). Patients score scar colour, pliability, thickness, relief, itching and pain, while the observer scores scar vascularisation, pigmentation, pliability, thickness and relief (*Table 2*).

This scale was compared with the more established VSS and was found to be more consistent and reliable (Draaijers et al., 2004). However, this was a small study of 20 patients with a total of 49 scars. Since the patients rated more than one scar on their body, the ratings may not have been independent of each other. The authors recognised this as a possible cause of bias.

A further study of the patient and observer scar assessment scale reported good internal consistency, reliability and agreement. Three independent observers used the scale to assess 100 linear scars, while the patients simultaneously evaluated their scars. A single observer reliably evaluated the scars with respect to total scores ($r=0.088$, $p<0.001$), indicating good feasibility for clinical follow-up and research purposes (Van de Kar et al., 2005).

Based on this, the patient and observer scar assessment scale appears to be the most suitable subjective scar evaluation tool, although further refinements may be possible. For instance, the number of parameters in the patient scale may be reduced. However, this can be done only after more experience with the scale as the relevance of each parameter needs to be evaluated for different scar categories in different patient groups (Van de Kar et al., 2005).

Objective scar assessment

Aspects of a scar that can be objectively measured are its structural, mechanical, microscopic and physiologic characteristics (Powers et al, 1999). Its physical characteristics such as size, shape (area), volume (depth x height), colour, texture and pliability can also be measured.

Table 2. Patient and Observer Scar Assessment Scale

Patient scar assessment scale

No, no complaints	1	2	3	4	5	6	7	8	9	10	Yes, worst imaginable
Is the scar painful?	O	O	O	O	O	O	O	O	O	O	
Is the scar itching?	O	O	O	O	O	O	O	O	O	O	

No, as normal skin	1	2	3	4	5	6	7	8	9	10	Yes, very different
Is the colour of the scar different?	O	O	O	O	O	O	O	O	O	O	
Is the scar more stiff?	O	O	O	O	O	O	O	O	O	O	
Is the thickness of the scar different?	O	O	O	O	O	O	O	O	O	O	
Is the scar irregular?	O	O	O	O	O	O	O	O	O	O	

Observer scar assessment

Normal skin	1	2	3	4	5	6	7	8	9	10	Worst scar imaginable
Vascularisation	O	O	O	O	O	O	O	O	O	O	
Pigmentation	O	O	O	O	O	O	O	O	O	O	Hypo Mix Hyper
Thickness	O	O	O	O	O	O	O	O	O	O	
Relief	O	O	O	O	O	O	O	O	O	O	
Pliability	O	O	O	O	O	O	O	O	O	O	

Scar dimension

It is difficult to determine the size, shape and area of a scar because the margins can be irregular, the scar rounded rather than flat, and the surface curved. Tracing scar margins on clear plastic film or planimetry by photography are the two most common methods used (Oliveira et al., 2005). More sophisticated techniques involve digitally tracing the scar margin and using a computer to calculate the surface area. However, Van Zuijlen et al. (2001) found that, in some burn scars, the margins became blurred and so digital planimetry analysis was not possible in all cases.

Newer three-dimensional techniques show promise of being an accurate and reliable method of objectively assessing the physical qualities of a scar. Taylor et al. (2007) successfully used a non-contact, three-dimensional digitiser to reliably estimate the dimensions of keloid scars. With further development, this might become the 'gold standard'. However, due to its expense, size and the need for further evaluation, at present this is a research tool rather than a device that can be used in a clinical setting.

Scar volume/thickness

Measuring scar volume requires determination of the thickness of the scar, which may protrude from the surface in an irregular way or extend below it. An important question is whether we are interested in the total thickness of the scar or only the protruding part above the skin surface (Van Zuijlen et al., 2002).

When assessing scar thickness above the skin surface, the VSS measures scar height, although the method is rather subjective. Nedelec et al. (2000) described how dental elastomer putty casts were made to objectively measure surface volume, but this is impractical and time-consuming .

Ultrasound has been used to provide quantitative data on scar thickness above and below the skin surface and to monitor scar treatments (Humbleton et al., 1992; Fong et al, 1997).

Again, the most promising technique to date for measuring scar volume is three-dimensional imaging. So far, only small studies have been performed and further evaluation is recommended before this technique can be adopted (Taylor et al, 2007).

Scar colour

The colour of a scar is affected by two main factors: its pigmentation and vascularity. While these are VSS parameters, there was only moderate interrater agreement for them (k=0.5) (Sullivan et al, 1990). As a result, in their Manchester scar scale, Beausang et al. (1998) proposed that pigmentation and vascularity should not be rated separately, but that instead any colour mismatch shoud be ranked as none, slight, obvious or gross mismatch (*Table 3*). By doing this, their overall scale achieved a better correlation ($r=0.87$). However, these remain subjective evaluations.

For objective colour data, devices such as the DermaSpectrometer (Cyberderm, US), Chromameter (Minolta, Japan) and Mexameter (Courage + Khazaka, Germany) have been applied to scar evaluation (Oliviera et

---

Table 3. Manchester scar scale

Visual analogue scale

Colour

    Perfect = 1
    Slight mismatch = 2
    Obvious mismatch = 3
    Gross mismatch = 4

Matt = 1, shiny = 2

Contour

    Flush with surrounding skin = 1
    Slightly proud / indented = 2
    Hypertrophic = 3
    Keloid = 4

Distortion

    None = 1
    Mild = 2
    Moderate = 3
    Severe = 4

Texture

    Normal = 1
    Just palpable = 2
    Firm = 3
    Hard = 4

---

al., 2005; Kim et al., 2006). The DermaSpectrometer and Mexameter are based on spectrophotometric colour measurement, which calculates an erythema and melanin index.

Oliveria et al. (2005) compared the DermaSpectrometer and Chromameter with the VSS on 69 patients with burn scars between six months and two years after injury. The DermaSpectrometer had the best correlation with the VSS for colour ($p<0.05$) and pigmentation ($p<0.01$). The Chromameter, however, failed to differentiate between normal and red ($p>0.05$) and hypo- and hyperpigmented scars ($p=0.28$).

Kim et al. (2006) used the Mexameter to objectively evaluate the natural change in erythema and pigmentation of split-thickness skin graft scars. They reported this provided reproducible estimates of haemoglobin and melanin content of the skin graft, but did not present any evidence to substantiate this. Since they did not correlate the Mexameter measurements with the clinical appearance of the skin graft, it is impossible to comment on the validity of the device.

Further studies are required, and it is still unclear which colour measurement tool is most accurate.

Scar pliability

Pliability is an important aspect of a scar, but it is difficult to define and measure (Powers et al., 1999). Its importance was highlighted by Truong et al., (2005) who found that patients' overall satisfaction was significantly associated with self-ratings of scar pliability ($p<0.001$), while age, type of surgery, time after surgery, scar location, scar length, VSS score, and patient rating of colour were not significant ($p>0.05$).

Pliability includes the elasticity of the scar, which is determined in part by its tensile characteristics. Mechanical instruments divide the pliability of the skin into elastic and viscous segments that correspond directly with rapid stretch and slow stretch. They measure both skin deformation during loading and recovery after release of the load (Boyce et al., 2000). Various devices use different types of loading, which can be categorised as torsion, pressure or suction.

Torsion devices

Devices that assess torsional forces cause a load in the horizontal plane instead of the plane perpendicular to the skin. The Dermal Torque Meter

(Diastron, Andover, UK) has been used to evaluate burn scars (Boyce et al., 2000). A flat 2cm rotating disk is placed in direct contact with the skin surface. A motor applies a rotational force to create a torque, to produce a time deformation curve.

Boyce et al. (2000) used the device to compare skin pliability of a cultured skin substitute and autograft, with normal controls. However, the study group comprised children (mean age 5.6 years) and the control group adults. The two are not comparable because the elastic properties of human skin differs with age, and burns in children have a greater tendency to hypertrophic scarring (Cua et al., 1990; Sheridan et al, 1994). As a result of this flaw, the study was unable to determine the suitability of the device.

Pressure devices

The Pneumatonometer (Solan model 30 classic, Medtronic, US) and the Durometer (Rex Gauge, US) use pressure to objectively measure skin pliability; both have been tested on burn scars (Oliveira et al., 2005).

The Pneumatonometer comprises an air-flow system, a sensor and a membrane that comes into direct contact with the skin surface. When applied, the amount of pressure needed to lock the system is measured (Spann et al., 1996).

The Durometer, which was originally developed to test the hardness of metals and plastics, applies an indentation load in the vertical direction on the specimen, and was first used on skin to assess scleroderma (Falanga and Bucalo, 1993).

Oliveria et al.'s (2005) study on 69 burn scars found that both devices correlated well with the VSS pliability score but the investigators preferred the Durometer because it was easier to use due to its smaller size. They concluded that the device was validated for use in all scar assessment. However, this should be viewed with caution as the Durometer may not be applicable to all scar locations. Previously, Falanga and Bucalo (1993) found that, where bony structures are situated directly under skin (ie, fingers, hand and face), the hardness of the bone influenced the Durometer measurement. Oliveria et al. (2005) measured thigh scars only. In addition, this was the first study in which the Durometer was used to evaluate scar hardness. Further assessment is required before this device can be widely adopted for objective scar assessment in all anatomical sites.

Suction devices

Suction methods aim to measure skin elevation caused by a controlled negative pressure over a defined area of skin, to create a derfomation over time curve (Gniadecka and Serup, 1995). In clinical trials two devices, the Cutometer (Courage + Khazaka, Germany) and the Dermafex (Cortex Technology, Denmark), were used to measure skin elasticity. However, only the Cutometer has been used in scar assessment. It has been reliably used to evaluate burns scars, dermal skin substitutes, split-skin grafts, donor sites and following reconstructive surgery (Van Zuijlen et al., 2002; Wisser et al., 2004; Oliviera et al., 2005; Kim et al., 2006; Rennekampff et al., 2006; Taylor et al., 2007).

Non-contact methods

Although most effort has been made to measure scar elasticity directly using contact devices, non-contact methods that can infer scar elasticity from observed tissue motion is an alternative option (Zhang et al., 2004).

A promising non-contact method of evaluating skin deformation is finite element modelling. This technique divides the object into a grid of small triangular or square elements, and the deformation of these elements under external forces are then modelled using basic laws of biomechanical physics (Tsap et al., 1998).

In a small study of four patients Zhang et al. (2004) created a finite element model based on natural image features and an adaptive mesh to estimate the relative elasticity of scars. Their model correlated well with the physicians' rating of the scar.

This method is still in the early experimental stages, but it may offer an elegant solution to the evaluation of the physical properties of scars and warrants further investigation.

Conclusion

Scar assessment has been overlooked in the past as the focus was to ensure that patients survive severe injuries. However, with improved survival it has become increasingly important to look at outcomes. Scarring may have long-lasting functional, cosmetic and psychological consequences for the patient.

The VSS was the first tool to attempt standardisation of scar assessment. Since then it has been recognised that, irrespective of the actual nature of the scar, the way in which the patient assesses the scar is important and can influence outcome and quality of life. Therefore, modifications to the VSS have been made (Baryza and Baryza, 1995; Yeong et al., 1997) and new tools developed such as the patient and observer scar assessment scale (Draaijers et al., 2004). However, subjective scar assessment tools have their limitations. An ideal scar assessment should try to include both objective and subjective aspects of a scar. A holistic approach would involve using subjective scales and objective tools in tandem. Hence, there has been a drive to develop devices to measure the objective aspects of a scar.

With advances in technology, techniques such three-dimensional scanning and finite element modelling show great promise. However, the use of instruments for assessment should not be considered inherently valid simply because they are objective. Data collected from devices represent a small fraction of the scar field, and not the entire scar area, so may not truly reflect the scar character. Therefore, without proper attention to these factors, sources of error may be introduced that can compromise the validity of the data. Hence, careful consideration and qualification is needed before we extrapolate biomechanical data to anatomic and physiological properties of skin. These should be tested rigorously with respects to concepts of reliability, reproducibility and validity.

References

Baryza MJ, Baryza GA (1995) The Vancouver Scar Scale: an administration tool and its interrater reliability. *J Burn Care Rehabil* **16**: 535–8

Beausang E, Floyd H, Dunn KW.et al. (1998) A new quantitative scale for clinical scar assessment. *Plast Reconstr Surg* **102**: 1954–61

Boyce ST, Supp AP, Wickett RR et al. (2000) Assessment with the dermal torque meter of skin pliability after treatment of burns with cultured skin substitutes. *J Burn Care Rehabil* **21**(1): 55–63

Brennan P, Silman A (1992) Statistical methods for assessing observer variability in clinical measures. *Br Med J* **304**: 1491

Crombie I (1996) *The pocket Guide to Critical Appraisal* (10th edn). London: BMJ

Cua AB, Wilhelm KP, Maibach HI (1990) Elastic properties of human skin: relation to age, sex, and anatomical region. *Arch Dermatol Res* **282**: 283–8

Draaijers L, Templeman F, Botman Y et al. (2004) The patient and observer scar assessment scale: a reliable and feasible tool for scar evaluation. *Plastic Reconstr Surg* **113**(7): 1960–5

Falanga V, Bucalo B (1993) Use of the durometer to assess skin hardness. *J Am Acad Dermatol* **29**(1): 47–51

Fong S, Hung L, Cheng J (1997) The cutometer and ultrasonography in the assessment of post burn hypertrophic scar: a preliminary study. *Burns* **23**(1): S12–S18

Gniadecka M, Serup J (1995) Suction chamber method for measurement of skin mechanical properties: the Dermaflex. In: Serup J, Jemec GBE (eds) *Handbook of Non-invasive Methods and the Skin.* CRC Press

Humbleton J, Shakespeare PG, Pratt BJ (1992) The progress of hypertrophic scars monitored by ultrasound measurements of thickness. *Burns* **18**: 301–07

Kim YJ, Kim MY, Lee PK et al. (2006) Evaluation of natural change of skin function in split thickness skin grafts by noninvasive bioengineering methods. *Dermatol Surg* 32: 1358–63

Martin D, Umraw N, Gomez M, Cartotto R (2003) Changes in subjective vs objective burn scar assessment over time: does the patient agree with what we think? *J Burn Care Rehabil* **24**(4): 239–44

Nedelec B, Shankowsky HA, Tredget EE (2000) Rating the resolving hypertrophic scar: comparison of the Vancouver Scar Scale and Scar volume. *J Burn Care Rehabil* **21**: 205–12

Oliveira GV, Chinkes D, Mitchell C et al. (2005) Objective assessment of burn scar vascularity, erythema, pliability, thickness and planimetry. *Dermatol Surg* **31**(1): 48–58

Powers P, Sarkar S, Goldof D et al. (1999) Scar assessment: current problems and future solutions. *J Burn Care Rehabil* **20**(1): 54–60

Rennekampff HO, Rabbels J, Reinhard V et al. (2006) Comparing the Vancouver Scar Scale with the cutometer in the assessment of donor site wounds treated with various dressings in a randomised trial. *J Burn Care Res* **27**(3): 345–51

Sheridan RL, Hegarty M, Tompkins RG, Burke JF (1994) Artificial skin in massive burns: results to ten years. *Eur J Plastic Sur* **17**: 91–3

Spann K, Mileski WJ, Atiles L et al. (1996) Use of a pneumatonometer in burn scar assessment. J *Burn Care Rehabil* **17**: 515–17

Streiner DL, Norman GR (1989) *Health measurement scales: a practical guide to their development and use.* Oxford: Oxford University Press

Sullivan T, Smith J, Kermode J et al. (1990) Rating the burn scar. *J Burn Care Rehabil* **11**: 256–60

Taylor B, McGrouther DA, Bayat A (2007) Use of a non contact 3D digitiser to measure the volume of kelod scars: a useful tool for scar assessment. *J Plast Reconstr Aesthet Surg* **60**: 87–94

Truong PT, Abnousis F, Yong CM et al. (2005) Standardized assessment of breast cancer surgical scars integrating the Vancouver Scar Scale, short form McGill pain questionnaire, and patients' perspectives. *Plastic Reconstr Surg* **116**(5): 1291–9

Tsap LV, Goldgof DB, Sarkar S, Powers PS (1998) A vision based technique for objective assessment of scars. *IEEE Transactions Medical Imaging* **17**(4): 620–33

Van de Kar A, Corion L, Smeulders M et al. (2005) Reliable and feasible evaluation of linear scars by the Patient and Observer Scar Assessment Scale. *Plastic Reconstr Surg* **116**(2): 514–22

Van Zuijlen PP, Angeles AP, Kreis RW et al. (2002) Scar assessment tools: implications for current research. *Plast Reconstr Surg* **109**(3): 1108–22

Van Zuijlen P, Vloemans J, van Trier A et al. (2001) Dermal substitute in acute burns and reconstructive surgery: a subjective and objective long term follow up. *Plast Reconstr Surg* **108**: 1938–46

Wisser D, Rennekampff HO, Schallere HE (2004) Skin assessment of burn wounds covered with a collagen based dermal substitute in a 2 year follow-up. *Burns* **30**: 399–401

Yeong EK, Mann R, Engrav LH et al. (1997) Improved burn scar assessment with use of a new scar rating scale. *J Burn Care Rehabil* **18**(4): 353–5

Zhang Y, Goldof DB, Sarkar S, Tsap L (2004) A modelling approach for burn scar assessment using natural features and elastic property. *IEEE Trans Med Imaging* **23**(10): 1325–9

CHAPTER 3

Evaluation of pH measurement as a method of wound assessment

V K Shukla, D Shukla, S K Tiwary, S Agrawal and A Rastogi

Wound healing is a complex process, so it is important to have an objective measure of healing status. Ideally, such a measure would be simple, accessible, sensitive, precise, reproducible and cause minimal or no discomfort to the patient. One option might involve determining the wound pH. Lengheden and Jansson's *in vitro* study into the effect of pH on fibroblast repopulation showed that wound cell migration and DNA synthesis decreased as the pH increased (Lengheden and Jansson, 1995).

Under normal circumstances, as first described by Hesus et al. in 1892 and Schade and Marchionini in 1928, an acidic milieu is found on the skin surface. This varies between pH 4 and pH 6, depending on the anatomical location and the person's age.

The acidic milieu is an important aspect of the skin's barrier function and appears to protect against external chemicals (Dikstein and Zlotogorski, 1994; Rippke et al., 2002).

The pH value within the wound milieu directly and indirectly influences all of the biochemical reactions that take place during the healing process. Interestingly, so far it has been a neglected outcome parameter (Schneider et al., 2007).

The skin's acidic milieu is disturbed in wounds, where underlying tissue with a pH milieu of 7.4 becomes exposed. Most relevant human pathogenic bacteria need pH values above 6, and their growth is inhibited by a lower pH value (O'Meara et al., 2000 ; Stewart et al., 2002). Stüttgen and Schaefer (1974) showed that bacterial colonisation causes the pH milieu of normal skin to become more alkaline.

Restoring the natural acidic milieu on the skin can thus help to reduce the microbial load on the body surface, even if such microbes are antibiotic-resistant. An interventional clinical study supported this by showing that topical application of acidic ointments in patients with diabetes and stroke significantly reduced the bacterial load on their skin surface (Kurabayaski et al., 2002). It is interesting and somewhat paradoxical that the activity of essential bacterial enzymes, such as most Staphylococci-derived proteases, is diminished in an alkaline milieu, whereas the acidic pH on normal skin promotes greater protease activity (Glinz, 1971).

Acidic wound fluid has been found to be associated with rapid wound healing (Lengheden and Jansson, 1995). Changing the wound environment from alkaline to acidic has been shown to accelerate healing (Lengheden and Jansson, 1995). Indeed, non-permeable hydrocolloid dressings are used to modify the wound environment to an acidic pH and so retard bacterial growth and promote wound healing (Schneider et al., 2007). The same is true of povidone-iodine, Dakin's solution and acetic acid (Schneider et al., 2007).

This study aimed to assess variations in pH levels in wounds and explore the relationship between wound pH and the state of healing.

Method

Fifty consecutive patients with acute or chronic wounds attending the wound clinic at University Hospital, Varanasi, India, had the pH of their wounds measured with litmus pH paper strips (gradations of 0.5, ranging from 6.5 to 9). The accuracy of the litmus strips was confirmed by testing against standard solutions of known pH.

There were no exclusion criteria other than malignant wounds, osteomyelitis and patient unwillingness to attend the clinic regularly for treatment and follow-up assessment.

Informed consent was obtained from the patients, and ethical approval was obtained from the institute's ethics committee.

The mean wound duration was 16 ± 3 weeks (range 3–28). Patients had used a number of different topical medications (neomycin, povidone-iodine, mupirocin, silver sulphadiazine and herbal preparations) before attending the clinic. Seven patients (14%) had diabetes, two had leprosy (4%), one had tuberculosis (2%) and one had chronic venous insufficiency (2%).

Wound sizes were as follows:

- Less than 4cm² in 15 patients (30%)
- 4–10cm² in 25 patients (50%)
- Greater than 10cm² in 10 patients (20%).

At baseline most wounds (94%) were characterised by the presence of slough, pus or copious discharge. The exudate level was reflected by the number of gauze dressing changes required, which ranged from four to 18 per day.

Sharp debridement and cleansing with normal saline were undertaken at the first visit. The litmus paper strip was then placed on the wound bed for five seconds, removed and, 30 seconds later, compared with the colour code. Saline would be unlikely to affect the outcome as it was used in all cases.

Wound dressings (saline-impregnated gauze) were changed daily (modern wound dressings were not available at the hospital). Wounds were irrigated with normal saline during the dressing change. All wounds were managed by the same protocol.

The wound condition ('unhealthy', 'granulating' or 'healing'), exudate level and pH were recorded on a weekly basis on days 1, 7 and 15. Acute wounds were classified as unhealthy if slough, pus or copious discharge were present. Chronic wounds were defined as unhealthy if slough was present. Wounds with pink granulation tissue were defined as granulating. Healing wounds had a sloping edge with epithelial ingrowth. Exudate from all wounds was tested for culture and sensitivity each week.

Paired samples *t*-tests were used to analyse differences in wound condition, discharge and pH between days 1 and 7 as well as days 7 and 15. Observations were subsequently analysed using the paired Student's *t*-test. All wounds were included in the analysis.

Results

Fifty patients (each with one wound) were enrolled into the study. The study group comprised 37 males (74%) and 13 females (26%), with a mean age of 48 ± 6 years (range 7–74).

Twenty-six wounds (52%) were classed as acute, and were caused by trauma (22%), cellulitis (16%) or an unknown cause (14%). Most of the traumatic injuries resulted from outdoor activities undertaken by the male population.

Twenty-four wounds (48%) were chronic and caused by trauma (26%), diabetes (14%), leprosy (4%), tuberculosis (2%) and chronic venous insufficiency (2%).

Most of the wounds (both chronic and acute) were located on the lower limbs (78%), followed by the trunk (12%), upper limb (6%) and face (4%).

Changes in the condition of the wound, discharge and pH are given in *Table 1*. On the first day 94% of the wounds were classified as unhealthy. The wound condition subsequently improved as 88% and 98% progressed to the granulating or healing categories on day 7 and day 15 respectively. A significant difference was found in the wound condition between days 1 and 7 ($p=0.00$) and between days 7 and 15 ($p=0.00$). This clearly shows that the wound condition improved during the study period.

Wound discharge was classified as purulent, serosanguineous, serous and absent, which roughly corresponds to the wound healing process. Wound discharge changed from purulent in most wounds (84%) on day 1 to serous and serosanguineous in 58% on day 7, and was serous or absent in 86% on day 15. Paired samples *t*-test showed there was no significant difference in wound discharge between days 1 and 7 ($p=0.883$), whereas there was a significant difference between days 7 and 15 ($p=0.00$) (*Table 2*). Clearly, in the first few days no significant difference was observed in wound discharge, but after seven days it significantly decreased.

Wound pH was greater than 8.5 in most patients on day 1 (94%), 8.0 to 9.0 in 88% on day 7 and less than 8.5 in 78% on day 15. There was

Table 1. Wound condition, discharge and pH on days 1, 7 and 15

	Day 1 No of patients (%)	Day 7 No of patients (%)	Day 15 No of patients (%)
Wound condition			
Unhealthy	47 (94)	6 (12)	1 (2)
Granulating	2 (4)	34 (68)	21 (42)
Healing	1 (2)	10 (20)	28 (56)
Wound discharge			
Purulent	42 (84)	18 (36)	0 (0)
Serosanguineous	2 (4)	15 (30)	7 (14)
Serous	6 (12)	14 (28)	13 (26)
Absent	0 (0)	3 (6)	30 (60)
Wound pH			
>9	27 (54)	5 (10)	0 (0)
8.5–9.0	20 (40)	24 (48)	13 (26)
8.0–8.5	3 (6)	20 (40)	13 (26)
7.5–8.0	0 (0)	1 (2)	17 (34)
<7.5	0 (0)	0 (0)	7 (14)

Table 2. Paired samples *t*-test results for wound conditions, discharge and pH between days 1 and 7 plus days 7 and 15

	t value	*p* value
Wound pH		
Day 1 versus day 7	13.25	0.000
Day 7 versus day 15	10.53	0.000
Wound discharge		
Day 1 versus day 7	0.148	0.883
Day 7 versus day 15	6.276	0.000
Wound conditions		
Day 1 versus day 7	12.374	0.000
Day 7 versus day 15	6.467	0.000

All results are significant except for wound discharge on day 1 versus day 7

Table 3. Wound culture and associated pH

Organisms	Approximate wound pH
Pseudomonas aeruginosa	>8.5
Escherichia coli, Klebsiella pneumoniae,	
Proteus	8.0
Staphylococcus aureus	7.5

a significant difference in the wound pH levels between days 1 and 7 (p=0.00) and between days 7 and 15 (p=0.00), indicating that there was a significant decrease in the wound pH during the study period (*Table 2*). Thus, progression of wound healing was associated with a decrease in wound pH.

Twenty-nine wounds (58%) were culture positive; common organisms cultured were *Escherichia coli, Klebsiella pneumoniae*, Proteus, *Pseudomonas aeruginosa* and *Staphylococcus aureus*. Results for wound culture and associated pH are given in *Table 3*. Systemic antibiotics were used in accordance with sensitivity.

Discussion

Major advances have been made in wound healing, with better understanding of the pathogenetic mechanisms involved. Current methods of wound assessment rely on subjective visual scoring (Krasner, 1997) and objective approaches which include area measurements, tracing and photography. A more precise approach is urgently needed. The objective approaches referred to above are used to make a diagnosis, confirm efficacy of clinical management and predict treatment options. Assessment methods need to be reproducible, so they can also be performed by technicians and sent via telemedicine for expert evaluation. Various parameters, such as measurement of colour, pH, temperature, tissue perfusion, malodour, area and volume of the wound bed, have been investigated (Menke et al., 2007).

A study on chronic venous leg ulcers and pressure ulcers found that the wound-bed pH was alkaline or neutral when compared with the intact surrounding skin (Glibbery and Mani, 1992). This changed depending on the ulcer grade, becoming acidic during epithelialisation (Tsukada et al., 1992).

Similar studies have shown that wound pH is important during the healing of chronic wounds, with prolonged acidification increasing the healing rate in chronic venous leg ulcers (Wilson et al., 1979).

In our study 58% wounds were culture positive, and an association was found between the type of organism and wound pH (*Table 3*). Another study demonstrated that the optimal pH of granulation tissue in a burn wound for graft take was 7.2–7.5 and was related to the quantity and species of bacteria present (Chai, 1992).

Varghese et al. (1986) found that wound fluid was more acidic under a non-permeable hydrocolloid dressing than an oxygen-permeable polyurethane one; bacterial growth studied *in vitro* was retarded at a more acidic pH, with a similar rate to that found under the hydrocolloid dressing. Therefore, dressings that decrease the wound pH provide an optimum environment for normal repair and regeneration.

Protease activity is strongly dependent on the pH of its surroundings (Schultz et al., 2005). Open wounds tend to have a neutral or alkaline pH, predominantly in the range of 6.5–8.5 (Dissemond et al., 2003). Since chronic wounds have permanently elevated protease levels, resulting in a prolonged inflammatory state, one strategy to promote healing might be to use a pH modulator to decrease proteolytic activity to the normal levels observed in acute wounds (post-48 hours). A weak acidic environment may promote healing in open wounds by inhibiting protease activity (Leveen et al., 1973).

Lowering wound pH to around 5 dramatically slows down the activity of harmful proteases, which can break down the newly formed matrix and prolong inflammation (Greener et al., 2005). Lowering the pH from 8 to 4 can reduce protease activity by 80% (Schultz et al., 2005). Greener et al. (2005) stated that wound pH must be greater than 4 for healing to take place and less than 7 to avoid degradation of the newly formed matrix.

The wound environment can be modified by changing the pH to promote healing in both acute and chronic wounds, which are serious problems for both patients and practitioners (Tiwary et al., 2006). Investigations looking at various aspects of wound healing have supported the view that an acidic pH in the wound supports most aspects of the natural healing process. Such a pH milieu suppresses bacterial growth, reduces proteolytic activity, enhances fibroblast growth *in vitro*, increases oxygen supply and is an indicator of successful self-healing of chronic wounds (Schneider et al., 2007). Different absorbents (Curasorb, Tyco; Cadesorb, Smith & Nephew; Sorbsan, Unomedical) have been used to control moisture levels in the wound, alter the local wound environment and decrease the wound pH to promote healing. Cadesorb consists of a cross-linked starch matrix which neutralises excess basic ions present by exchanging them with H+ ions. This lowers the pH, in turn inhibiting protease activity (Schneider et al., 2007).

Study limitations include the inclusion of both acute and chronic wounds in the same study, that randomisation was done irrespective of the wound duration, and the focus on wound-surface pH alone, which may or may not reflect wound-tissue pH. Furthermore, dressing changes, the use of different types of dressings and exposure to air during dressing changes might alter the local wound environment and pH.

Conclusion

Wound pH measurements, which can be obtained efficiently and non-invasively with no discomfort to the patient, can provide important information, particularly during wound bed preparation where the microbiological profile is crucial for complete wound healing. The use of pH measurements in wound evaluation will help provide an objective measure of the wound condition and thus help facilitate wound healing.

References

Chai JK (1992) The pH value of granulating wound and skin graft in burn patients (in Chinese). *Zhonghua Zheng Xing Shao Shang Wai Ke Za Zhi* **8**(3): 177–178, 246

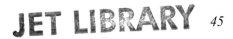

Dikstein S, Zlotogorski A (1994) Measurement of skin pH. *Acta Derm Venereol Suppl* **185**: 18–20

Dissemond J, Witthoff M, Brauns TC et al. (2003) pH values in chronic wounds: evaluation during modern wound therapy. *Hautarzt* **54**(10): 959–65

Glibbery A, Mani R (1992) pH measurements in leg ulcers. *Int J Microcirc Clin Exptl* **109** (Suppl).

Glinz W (1971) pH-Mesungen des Granulationsgewebes vor freier Hauttransplantation. *Zentralbl Phlebol* **10**: 105–13

Greener B, Hughes AA, Bannister NP et al. (2005) Proteases and pH in chronic wounds. *J Wound Care* **14**(2) 59–61

Hesus E (1892) Die Reaktion des Schweißes beim gesunden Menschen. *Monatsschr Prakt Dermatol* **343**: 400–1

Krasner D (1997) Wound healing scale, version 1.0: a proposal. *Adv Wound Care* **10**: 82–5

Kurabayashi H, Tamura K, Machida I et al. (2002) Inhibiting bacteria and skin pH in hemiplegia: effects of washing hands with acidic mineral water. *Am J Phys Med Rehabil* **81**: 40–6

Lengheden A, Jansson L (1995) pH effects on experimental wound healing of human fibroblasts in vitro. *Eur J Oral Sci* **103**(3): 148–55

Leveen HH, Falk G, Borek B et al. (1973) Chemical acidification of wounds: an adjuvant to healing and the unfavorable action of alkalinity and ammonia. *Ann Surg* **178**(6): 745–53 Menke NB, Ward KR, Tarynn MW et al. (2007) Impaired wound healing. *Clin Dermatol* **25**: 19–25

O'Meara S, Cullum N, Majid M et al. (2000) Systemic review of wound care management: (3) antimicrobial agents for chronic wounds; (4) diabetic foot ulceration. *Health Technol Assess* **4**: 1–237

Rippke F, Schreiner V, Schwanitz HJ (2002) The acidic milieu of the horny layer: new findings on the physiology and pathophysiology of skin pH. *Am J Clin Dermatol* **3**: 261–72

Schade H, Marchionini A (1928) Der Säuremantel der Haut. *Klin Wochenschr* **7**: 12–24

Schneider LA, Korber A, Grabbe S et al. (2007) Influence of pH on wound-healing: a new perspective for wound-therapy? *Arch Dermatol Res* **298**: 413–20

Schultz GS, Mozingo D, Romanelli M et al. (2005) Wound healing and TIME: new concepts and scientific application. *Wound Repair Regen* **13**(4): SI–SII Stewart CM, Cole MB, Legan JD et al. (2002) Staphylococcus aureus growth boundaries: moving towards mechanistic predictive models based on solute-specific effects. *Appl Environ Microbiol* **68**: 1864–71

Stüttgen G, Schaefer H (1974) Die Hautoberfläche. In: Stüttgen G., Schaefer H. (eds) *Funktionelle Dermatologie*. Springer

Tiwary SK, Shukla D, Tripathi AK et al. (2006) Effect of placental extract-gel and cream on non-healing wounds. *J Wound Care* **15**: 325–28 Tsukada K, Tokunaga K, Iwama T et al. (1992) The pH changes of pressure ulcers related to the healing process of wounds. *Wounds* **4**(1): 16–20

Varghese MC, Balin AK, Carter DM et al. (1986) Local environment of chronic wounds under synthetic dressings. *Arch Dermatol* **122**: 1 52–7 Wilson IAI, Henry M, Quill RD et al. (1979) The pH of varicose ulcer surfaces and its relationship to healing. *VASA* **8**: 339–42

The potential effect of fibroblast senescence on wound healing and the chronic wound environment

E A Henderson

The human body ages as a result of failure in the replication cycle of cells, otherwise known as cell senescence (Hayflick, 1965). In humans, cell senescence is thought to prevent genetic mutations and disease, but has the side-effect of organismic ageing (Campisi, 1996). All replicating cells senesce, but this occurs heterogeneously across the cell population, where the structure and biochemical make-up is altered (Stephens et al., 2003). This review focuses on the fibroblast cell as senescence has been shown to have several effects on its function, including reduction in number and size and decreased mobility and proliferation (Brown, 2004). As the fibroblast plays a key role in wound healing by initiating the proliferative phase and mediating remodelling (Leaper and Harding, 1998), failure of this mechanism could lead to failure of healing.

Telomere-dependent shortening

Telomeres are stretches of repetitive DNA with high G–C strand symmetry that 'cap' the chromosome ends (Von Zglinicki, 2002) and are thought to provide the cell replication counting mechanism, or 'biological clock'. With each replication (population doubling), the cell chromosomal ends (or telomeres) become progressively shorter until they are critically short and unable to replicate further (Smith and Pereira-Smith, 1996). This is thought to occur in all normal animal cells, except some stem cells (Smith and Kipling, 2004).

Many authors (Takai et al., 2003; Zou et al., 2004; Von Zglinicki et al., 1995, 2005) now consider the DNA damage response to be the primary trigger of telomere-dependent replicative senescence. This damage response occurs when uncapping of the shortened telomere causes chromosome instability, which exposes double strand breaks in need of repair. This in turn initiates a signalling pathway that results in the formation of p53, a protein responsible for controlling senescence, preventing replication occurring in potentially DNA-damaged chromosomes (Smith and Kipling, 2004).

The function of p53 is multiple and complex and not yet fully understood, but Seluanov et al. (2001) found it was modified in senescent cells, in which apoptosis was resisted and necrosis occurred instead, inducing inflammatory cells. However, this study is somewhat misleading as the conclusions are drawn from old fibroblast cells rather than senescent cells and no measure of the senescent cell phenotype was undertaken.

Smith and Pereira-Smith (1996) investigated the possibility of a DNA-damage response. They found that, when the telomere-protective protein TRF-2 was inhibited, senescence was induced in the presence of DNA-damage response factors Rad 17, H2AX and ATM, indicating that a DNA damage response does occur. These findings are, however, hard to decipher and validate as the article format is confusing with no clear methodology, aims or conclusions.

Zou et al. (2004) investigated whether specific short telomeres have a role in senescence or act as sentinels to monitor telomere shortening. One function of the telomere is to conceal the chromosome ends from identification as chromosome breaks in need of repair. When the chromosome becomes uncapped signal-free ends become exposed. Zou et al. (2004) found that specific telomeres with a high fraction of signal-free ends become localised to DNA-damage foci at the time of senescence, whereas telomeres with a low fraction of signal-free ends do not. This suggests that the most damaged telomere ends induce the DNA damage-signalling pathway that, in turn, affects other shortened but less damaged telomeres. This study recognised that telomere shortening is not a universal process but that the effects from the most damaged chromosomes have consequences for the whole cell. The authors suggested that the end associations, rather than the damage response, induces the senescent phenotype, but failed to argue this point effectively in their conclusions due to a lack of research evidence.

Zhang and Cohen (2004) investigated the role of Smad ubiquitination regulatory factor-2 (SMURF-2), an encoding gene for the TGF-β-signalling pathway, in activating telomere-dependent senescence. They found that SMURF-2 is regulated by progressive telomere shortening and is capable of producing the senescence phenotype in the absence of other factors previously mentioned.

This study was conducted using human fibroblast cells, one of the few cells that produce this gene. The authors suggested that replicative senescence may be induced and modulated by many different pathways in a given cell type at any given time, such as elevation of p21 protein or expression of human papilloma virus 16, E6 and E7 oncoproteins, and so cannot be attributed to a single cause.

The results must be appraised with caution, however, as the study is reported in a confusing format, making it difficult to follow the thought process to the conclusions. For example, the term 'telomere attrition' is used as a reference for their methodology but is not explained. Oxidative stress — cell damage caused by reactive oxygen species or free radical unpaired ions that are highly reactive and unstable — is excluded as an inducer of SMURF-2 but the dose or duration of exposure are not explained. Similarly, with DNA damage no markers were sought to ascertain if the stresses had an effect at a cellular level.

The use of viral oncoproteins or tumour-generating proteins to cause mutations in the cell-regulation pathways to induce senescence also affects the validity of the findings as these proteins have many sites of action, making it impossible to attribute the effects of their actions to one source (Smith and Kipling, 2004).

Martin-Ruiz et al. (2004) found that there was great heterogeneity in the population of fibroblasts they studied and that telomere length varied from cell to cell. Thus, cells do not age in a uniform fashion or senesce in a regimented way. The authors discussed how oxidative stress may be responsible for this finding. This study is presented in a logical way that lends confidence in the validity of the findings.

Betts et al. (2008), in a study using primary fetal bovine fibroblast cultures, demonstrated that, by lowering the oxygen content of the cell culture environment, the replicative lifespan of the fibroblasts was extended. Additional effects included a decrease in the rate of telomere shortening and a reduction in the incidence of chromosomal abnormalities

The implications from all these studies support the complexity of this process and the unlikelihood that the telomere functions purely as a biological clock.

Stress-induced senescence

Further studies have noted that senescence is induced via pathways that accelerate shortening of the telomere or cause DNA damage via telomere-independent mechanisms. Oxidative stress is caused by mitochondrial aerobic respiration, but with age, chronic disease and prolonged inflammation, such as in chronic wound healing, these mechanisms can become inefficient, resulting in oxidative damage to the cell. This is normally mopped up by a variety of intra- and extracellular mechanisms. Von Zglinicki et al. (1995) found that mild oxidative stress irreversibly blocks proliferation of fibroblasts *in vitro* and that the effects depend on the length of the telomere rather than the population-doubling level. These findings are plausible given the clear methodology and research design.

Chen et al. (2004) demonstrated mutations in experimental groups that are associated with increased longevity are attributed to their antioxidant abilities. This study supports the findings of Von Zglinicki (2002) that hyperoxic cells display all the phenotypic changes of senescence including morphological changes and telomere length and that senescence was induced after repeated exposure to oxidative stress. Chen et al. (2004) mentioned the role of naturally occurring antioxidant enzymes, superoxide dismutase-1 (SOD-1) and catalase, and that they are not present in senescent cells. As yet, there are few studies into the role of these antioxidants.

Samper et al. (2003) investigated mitochondrial oxidative stress in mouse embryos. They examined the natural antioxidant enzyme SOD-2 and found poor cell growth, increased cell death and increased chromosome damage in SOD-2 null mice. While it is impossible to directly apply these results to the human model, they support the significance of antioxidant mechanisms in preventing telomere damage.

A similar investigation by Busuttil et al. (2003) into murine mutations in high oxygen concentration found that the mutations led to an increased rate of immortalisation (ability to replicate without limitation) in the cells. They also discussed the importance of oxygen concentrations under experimental conditions on the cell types used. Different cell types and species have different tolerances to oxygen that can give skewed results if not taken into account in the analysis.

The prominent researcher Von Zglinicki (2002) theorised that telomere shortening and stress-induced damage are inexorably linked. The research supported the notion that oxidative stress increases damage on the telomere and that senescence is induced to protect the cell from potential mutations resulting from genome damage. Application of this theory (Von Zglinicki, 2002) concurs with the research evidence and offers the most credible explanation for this phenomenon.

There are several common flaws in the methodology of the *in vitro* studies that make direct application of these theories to the *in vivo* situation difficult. Many of the studies were carried out on cells that are animal in origin (Busuttil et al., 2003; Samper et al., 2003), particularly murine cells, which have very different characteristics to human cells, namely the expression of telomerase and ability to readily immortalise. Murine cells are much more susceptible to oxidative stress than human cells, making the culture method essential in maintaining reliability. Culture cells have been extracted at different stages of population doubling and from different cell populations such as lung fibroblasts, skin fibroblasts and neonatal cells. These variances make systematic review or meta-analyses of this experimental research impossible.

Furthermore, authors (Stephens et al., 2003; Takai et al., 2003; Von Zglinicki et al., 1995, 2005; Chen et al., 2004) used different cell biomarkers to recognise whether a senescent phenotype had been established. Few of these studies offer information on control groups, comparison or statistical analysis. Cell-culture media differ from study to study and are often made from cloned cells or cells that have been exposed to oncogenes, retroviruses and monoclonal antibodies, introducing many variables that are difficult to measure, control and understand. It is possible that the confounding variables in the methodologies alone could induce increased levels of senescence than would otherwise be found *in vivo*.

Upregulation of wound-healing mediators

Several authors (Saretzki et al., 1998; Shelton et al., 1999; Benanti et al., 2002) have found that, following DNA analysis of senescent cells, there was an upregulation of the transcription of several inflammatory mediators. These include pro-inflammatory cytokines, growth factors and proteases, with inherent implications of deregulation in the chronic wound environment.

Saretzki et al. (1998) compared gene expression in senescent cells and hyperoxic cells. They found increased expression of collagenase and matrix metalloproteinase-1 activity, but no difference in the synthesis of collagen I and III in young and old fibroblasts. Also noted was a high expression of plasminogen activator inhibitor (PAI-2).

These results concur with other studies on senescent cell type — increased transcription of proteinase is supported. However, the conclusion that proteinase activation is increased cannot be confirmed as it was not investigated in the research methodology.

Shelton et al. (1999) developed a DNA micro-array analysis system to identify gene expression in senescent cell types. They also found increased expression of inflammatory cytokines and matrix-modulating proteins but focused on the genetic expression of these factors and not activation and regulation.

Chronic wound cell senescence

Researchers have begun to investigate cellular senescence in chronic wounds, and studies have been carried out on venous leg ulcers and pressure ulcers but not diabetic foot ulcers.

Vande Berg et al. (1998) explored fibroblast senescence in pressure ulcers and concluded that it did not correlate with the age of the patient and there was great heterogeneity within the wound cell population. They also discovered that ulcer cells were capable of fewer population doublings than normal fibroblasts, regardless of patient age.

A further study by Vande Berg et al. (2005) of cultured fibroblasts from pressure ulcers *in vitro* found that there was a significant increase in plasmin and PAI produced by senescent ulcer fibroblasts and a non-significant increase in the production of transforming growth factor-beta (TGF-β).

The sample size in both studies is too small to be representative of the population, given the unaccounted confounding variables such as the ages of the donors or comorbidity. The authors suggested that the increases in these proteins are due to a chronic prolonged inflammatory response. This could be a result of senescence or conversely the cause of it.

Stephens et al. (2003) disputed these findings and found no evidence of cell senescence in chronic wound fibroblasts. This research differed from the previous studies because the cultures were from venous leg ulcers, and the exclusion criteria included patients with diabetes, compromised immune systems and infected wounds. The sample size once again was small and they used a collagen lattice to culture the cells. The cell culture samples were taken from the same site in the wound, thus not taking into account the heterogeneity of the cells. The cells were removed from the wound micro-environment and cultured in a sterile environment, possibly leading to an altered cell function *in vitro* (Kuhn et al., 2000), affecting the validity of the findings.

Until the cell culture medium is able to replicate the wound environment, it will be difficult to gain an accurate insight into the wound-cell function. It is difficult to compare the results of these studies due to their differing methodologies.

When Mendez et al. (1999) exposed neonatal skin fibroblasts to chronic venous ulcer fluid they found senescence was induced. The methodology does not explain whether cells were cultured in oxygen, and this is important given its potential adverse effects. They also found that endogenous cytokines interleukin-1 alpha (IL-1α), tumour necrosis factor-alpha (TNF-α) and TGF-β1 had an inhibitory effect on the neonatal fibroblast. This could be another mechanism of senescence that requires investigation as it may be induced by a cell-signalling pathway.

Moseley et al. (2004) investigating oxidative stress in acute and chronic wounds, concluded it was higher in chronic wounds, although this was not statistically significant. Chronic wounds exhibited significantly more antioxidant capability than acute wounds. This study was too small to be representative.

None of the studies discussed the intrinsic wound influences that could lead to an increased propensity to premature senescence of wound cells.

Conclusion

The chronic wound promotes an environment that generates high amounts of oxidative stress and pro-inflammatory cytokines which, in turn, will accelerate telomere degradation and cause alterations in cell signalling, resulting in premature senescence in cells with shortened telomeres. Although a wound may contain senescent cells, the entire cell population is not affected uniformly, which may affect the overall wound healing rate.

The discovery that there is an upregulation of inflammatory wound-healing factors adds another dimension to the implications of the senescence process, further complicating the healing process. As well as delaying skin closure, senescent cells may affect the mechanics and durability of the scar tissue. As yet no study has examined the senescent fibroblast and scarring.

The process of senescence remains poorly understood and more work needs to be undertaken into the role of receptors and signalling pathways and the implication of the natural antioxidant capabilities of cells.

Box 1. Summary of the main findings

ı Cell senescence is the phenomenon where a cell becomes unable to replicate and so is inactive. In humans this is thought to suppress tumour development

ı Cell senescence causes organismic ageing. The rate in which a cell reaches a senescent state depends on the length of the chromosome end (telomere)

ı The telomere helps the cell to replicate, stabilising and protecting this region of the chromosome end. With each replication, the telomere becomes shorter until it is critically short and in danger of 'uncapping' the chromosome end. At this point replication fails and senescence occurs (biological clock)

ı Senescence is induced via a DNA damage-response pathway when the telomere length becomes critically short

ı Studies have shown that naturally occurring and increased levels of oxidative stress, caused by inflammatory disease in cells, induces premature cell senescence

ı Senescent cells have been found in chronic wounds but not in the surrounding healthy skin. Chronic wound fluid has also been shown experimentally to induce senescence in otherwise healthy cells

---

In the future there may be a role for the application of topical antioxidants to chronic wounds, or gene therapy to induce increased production of cellular antioxidants. A further possible therapy is the use of gene therapy or topical induction of telomerase to immortalise senescent cell types. However, this therapy may have widespread negative effects such as inducing tumour development.

Clearly, further research needs to be conducted, particularly relating to wound healing. Further investigation of the *in vivo* wound environment may increase our understanding of this complex and dynamic process.

References

Benanti J, Williams D, Robinson K et al. (2002) Induction of extracellular matrix-remodelling genes by the senescence-associated protein APA-1. *Mol Cell Biol* **22**(21): 7385–97

Betts DH, Perrault SD, King WA (2008) Low oxygen delays fibroblast senescence despite shorter telomeres. *Biogerontology* **9**:19–31

Brown J (2004) The effects of ageing on fibroblast function during proliferation. *J Wound Care* **13**(3): 94–6

Busuttil R, Rubio M, Dolle M et al. (2003) Oxygen accelerates the accumulation of mutations during senescence and immortalization of murine cells in culture aging. *Cell* **2**: 287–94

Campisi J (1996) Replicative senescence: an old lives' tale? *Cell* **84**: 497–500

Chen J, Stoeber K, Kingsbury S et al. (2004) Loss of proliferative capacity and induction of senescence in oxidatively stressed human fibroblasts. *J Biol Chem* **279**(19): 49439–46

Hayflick L (1965) The limited *in vitro* lifetime of human diploid cell strains. *Exp Cell Res* **37**: 614–36

Kuhn A, Smith P, Hill D et al. (2000) *In vitro* populated collagen lattices are not good models of *in vivo* clinical wound healing. *Wound Repair Regen* **8**: 270–6

Leaper DJ, Harding KG (eds) (1998) *Wounds: Biology and Management.* Oxford: Oxford University Press

Martin-Ruiz C, Saretzki G, Petrie J et al. (2004) Stochastic variation in telomere shortening rate causes heterogeneity of human fibroblast replicative lifespan. *J Biol Chem* **279**(17): 17826–33

Mendez M, Rafetto J, Phillips T et al. (1999) The proliferative capacity of neonatal skin fibroblast is reduced after exposure to venous ulcer fluid: a potential mechanism for senescence in venous ulcers. *J Vasc Surg* **30**: 734–43

Moseley R, Hilton J, Waddington R et al. (2004) Comparison of oxidative stress biomarker profiles between acute and chronic wound environment. *Wound Repair Regen* **12**: 419–29.

Samper E, Nicholls D, Melov S (2003) Mitochondrial oxidative stress causes chromosomal instability of mouse embryonic fibroblasts aging. *Cell* **2**: 277–85

Saretzki G, Feng J, Von Zglinicki T, Villeponteau B (1998) Similar gene expression pattern in senescent and hyperoxic-treated fibroblasts. *J Gerontol* **53**(6): B438–42

Seluanov A, Gorbunova V, Falcovitz A et al. (2001) Change of death pathway in senescent human fibroblasts in response to DNA damage is caused by an inability to stabilize. *Mol Cell Biol* **21**(5): 1552–64

Shelton D, Chang E, Whittier P et al. (1999) Microarray analysis of replicative senescence. *Curr Biol* **9**(17): 939–45

Smith SK, Kipling D (2004) The role of replicative senescence in cancer and human ageing: utility (or otherwise) of murine models. *Cytogen Genome Res* **105**: 455–63

Smith JR, Pereira-Smith OM (1996) Replicative senescence: implications for *in vivo* aging and tumor suppression. *Science* **273**: 63–7

Stephens P, Cook H, Hilton J et al. (2003) An analysis of replicative senescence in dermal fibroblasts derived from chronic leg wounds predicts that telomerase therapy would fail to reverse their disease-specific cellular and proteolytic phenotyp. *Exp Cell Res* **283**: 22–35

Takai H, Smogorzewska A, de Lange T (2003) DNA damage foci at dysfunctional telomeres. *Curr Biol* **13**: 1549–56

Vande Berg J, Rose M, Haywood-Reid P et al. (2005) Cultured pressure ulcer fibroblasts show replicative senescence with elevated production of plasmin, plasminogen activator inhibitor-1, and transforming growth factor-beta1. *Wound Repair Regen* **13**: 76–83

Vande Berg J, Rudolph R, Hollan C, Haywood-Reid P (1998) Fibroblast senescence in pressure ulcers. *Wound Repair Regen* **6**(1): 38–49

Von Zglinicki T (2002) Oxidative stress shortens telomeres. *Trends Biochem Sci* **27**(7): 339–44

Von Zglinicki T, Saretzki G, Docke W, Lotze C (1995) Mild hyperoxia shortens telomeres and inhibits proliferation of fibroblasts: a model for senescence? *Exp Cell Res* **220**: 186–93

Von Zglinicki T, Saretzki G, Ladhoff J et al. (2005) Human cell senescence as a DNA damage response. *Mech Ageing Dev* **126**: 111–17

Zhang H, Cohen S (2004) Smurf-2 up-regulation activated telomere-dependent senescence. Genes Dev **18**: 3028–40

Zou Y, Sfeir A, Gryaznov S et al. (2004) Does a sentinel or a subset of short telomeres determine replicative senescence? *Mol Biol Cell* **15**: 3709–18

CHAPTER 5

Nitric oxide restores impaired healing in normoglycaemic diabetic rats

M Schäffer, M Bongartz, S Fischer, B Proksch and R Viebahn

Diabetes impairs wound healing (Goodson and Hunt, 1977; Falanga, 2005). The condition reduces the production of nitric oxide (Schaffer et al., 1997a; Witte et al., 2002a) a short-lived radical and biological mediator that plays an important role in wound repair (Schaffer et al., 1997a; Witte et al., 2002a). Supplemental L-arginine, the only physiological substrate for nitric-oxide synthesis, partially restores wound mechanical strength and collagen deposition (Witte et al., 2002b). *In vivo* application of a nitric-oxide donor has been shown to reverse the inhibitory effect of diabetic hyperglycaemia on wound repair (Witte et al., 2002a).

It is still unclear whether the diminished wound repair associated with diabetes is due to hyperglycaemia or other diabetes-related alterations in cellular immune function (Wetzler et al., 2000).

Deposition of collagen with subsequent cross-linking provides the principal strength characteristic of most wounds. In dermal wounds fibroblasts are the principal source of collagen. Regulation of wound-derived fibroblast collagen synthesis is mediated, in part, by nitric oxide in an autocrine and paracrine fashion (Schaffer et al., 1997b). The role of fibroblast nitric-oxide synthesis in diabetic healing has not been elucidated.

We hypothesised that nitric-oxide synthesis is impaired in wounds of normoglycaemic and hyperglycaemic diabetic rats, possibly reflecting the diminished fibroblast nitric-oxide synthesis and collagen production. Insulin treatment reverses the catabolic state of hyperglycaemia, leading to improved healing. Exogenous nitric oxide may further improve the outcome of impaired normoglycaemic diabetic healing.

Method

Animals

Twenty male genetically diabetic BioBreeding rats (Charles River, Sulzfeld, Germany), weighing between 220 and 250g, and 10 wild-type control rats (bred from Wistar rats) were caged in groups of two and given one week to acclimatise. The animals were fed a complete pelleted laboratory chow and had access to tap water ad libitum.

BioBreeding diabetes-prone rats spontaneously develop a form of diabetes that closely resembles human type 1 diabetes mellitus (Follak et al., 2004). Use of this model is well established in experimental bone fracture healing to investigate the impact of the diabetic state on repair mechanisms (Tyndall et al., 2003; Yang and Santamaria, 2006).

In our experiments, 10 diabetic rats received insulin implants (Linplants, LinShin Canada, Scarborough, Toronto, Canada) to render them normoglycaemic one week pre-wounding. The implants, which measured 7mm (length) x 2mm (diameter), released insulin (in microrecrystallised palmitic acid) at two units over 24 hours for 50 days.

The implants were inserted into the right abdominal region of anaesthetised rats (ketamine and xylazine at 100 and 15mg/kg body weight intraperitoneally respectively) using a trocar; no sutures were needed to hold the implants in place.

Within 24–72 hours, the rats with insulin implants had glucose levels of 90–120mg/dl. The control rats and the remaining 10 (hyperglycaemic) diabetic rats received vehicle implants.

All of the procedures used in the study were reviewed and approved by the local institutional animal care and use committee.

Wounding

Seven days following the insulin and vehicle implant application, all 30 rats underwent a 7cm dorsal skin incision under ketamine or xylazine anaesthesia (100 and 15mg/kg body weight intraperitoneally respectively) under aseptic conditions.

Ten pre-weighed, sterile, saline-moistened, polyvinyl alcohol sponges (Unipoint Industries, Thomasville, North Carolina, US) were inserted into subcutaneous pockets in each animal, and the wounds were closed with regular surgical staples. The animals were sacrificed 10 days post-wounding in order to harvest the sponges for subsequent analysis and fibroblast culture (Schaffer et al., 1997a, b).

Treatment with exogenous nitric oxide

In a separate experiment involving different animals, 10 insulin-treated diabetic BioBreeding rats and 10 non-insulin-treated diabetic BioBreeding rats received molsidomine (4mg/kg body weight per day) (Sigma, Munich, Germany), a nitric-oxide donor. The 10 control animals received a vehicle only (ethanol/water: 1/99 v/v).

The nitric-oxide treatment, which was administered by gavage (that is, given orally by oesophageal intubation using a blunt cannula) twice daily, started on the day of wounding.

With the exception of the use of the nitric-oxide donor, this experiment followed the same protocol as described above.

Assessment of wound healing

Wound-breaking strength

Following sacrifice 10 days post-wounding, the dorsal pelt containing the healing scar was removed and cut into seven equal strips (8mm wide) on a customised multiblade guillotine. Each strip was centred by a segment of the healing scar. Breaking strength was tested on a tensiometer (Zwick, Ulm, Germany) (Schaffer et al., 2002), using a constant speed of 50mm/minute. The force at which the strips broke was measured in Newtons (N).

Hydroxyproline

The two most cephalad-placed polyvinyl alcohol sponges were harvested, cleared of surrounding tissue and stored at –80°C for subsequent assay of hydroxyproline content, an index of reparative collagen deposition, using a colourimetrical method (Woessner, 1961; Schaffer et al., 2002). The values of the two sponges were averaged for each animal. The remaining sponges were retrieved for fibroblast culture and wound-cell analysis (Schaffer et al., 1997a).

Wound-fluid preparation

The remaining eight sponges from each animal were squeezed with forceps and the fluid recovered was centrifuged for 10 minutes (400 x g) and, subsequently, for 20 minutes (1600 x g) at 4°C for cell and debris removal. After filtering (0.45µm), the pooled wound fluid from each animal was stored at –80°C. Wound-fluid protein concentrations were determined by reaction with Coomassie blue, using the Bio-Rad Protein Assay Kit II (Bio-Rad Laboratories, Munich, Germany) (Schaffer et al., 2002).

Wound cell preparation

Two of the above squeezed sponges were cleared of surrounding granulation tissue. They were then minced with iris scissors in Dulbecco's Modified Eagle Medium (DMEM, Gibco, Grand Island, New York, US) containing 1% bovine serum albumin and passed through 80- and 100-mesh stainless steel screens. The recovered cells were combined with the cell pellet from wound-fluid preparation. Red blood cells were lysed with 0.83% ammonium chloride in (hydroxymethyl)-aminomethane hydrochloride (Tris) buffer (pH 7.4). Washed cells were counted using a Neubauer chamber and viability was checked by trypan blue exclusion (Schaffer et al., 1997a).

Fibroblast culture

The remaining six squeezed sponges were cleared of surrounding granulation tissue (Schaffer et al., 2002). Fibroblasts that had inflitrated the sponge were isolated by collagenase incubation (200U/ml, Sigma) and seeded in 75cm^2 tissue culture flasks in DMEM, supplemented with 10% foetal bovine serum (FBS). Cells were passaged weekly by trypsinisation and were used in experiments at the first passage. Data were recorded as the mean of triplicate cultures.

Synthesis of nitric oxide and collagen by fibroblasts

Viable (trypan blue dye exclusion), washed trypsinised fibroblasts (5 x105/500µl phenol red-free media) were plated in 24-well flat-bottomed tissue culture plates (Nunc, Naperville, Illinois) (Schaffer et al., 1997b, 2002).Viability of trypsinised fibroblasts was higher than 80% in all groups, with no significant differences between groups. This cell seeding concentration resulted in a confluent fibroblast population. No cell proliferation was detected on repeated DNA measurements during the 24-hour incubation period due to contact inhibition of confluent cells (data not shown).

Cell viability was routinely monitored by morphologic criteria and by measuring the release of intracellular lactate dehydrogenase (LDH-Toxicology kit, Sigma, St. Louis, Missouri, US).

At the end of the incubation, the plates were centrifuged for 10 minutes (400 x g) and the culture supernatants were removed and stored at –70°C for subsequent analysis of nitrite and hydroxyproline accumulation. Wells containing media alone were used as controls.

In these *in vitro* experiments, nitrite only was used as an index of nitric-oxide synthesis — nitrite accounts for more than 90% of total measurable nitrite and nitrate in cell culture supernatant (Schaffer et al., 2007b). Wound-derived fibroblasts spontaneously synthesise nitric oxide. Nitric-oxide synthesis, however, appears to be limited to the first and second passage post-harvest (Schaffer et al., 2007b). Cells were incubated in the presence or absence of the nitric-oxide donor S-nitroso-N-acetylpenicillamine (SNAP) (100μM).

Hydroxyproline content in cell supernatants was quantified using a colourimetrical method (Creemers et al., 1997). Briefly, culture supernatants were precipitated overnight at 4°C with absolute ethanol. Following centrifugation (1800g for 15 minutes at 4°C), supernatants were vacuum-evaporated, and the samples were hydrolysed for 3.5 hours at 135°C in 6N (normal) hydrogen chloride 60μl aliquots of dissolved (140μl demineralised water) and filtered (0.22μm) samples were used for final steps in a microtiter plate. After 20μl assay buffer and 40μl Chloramin-T were added, plates were incubated for 15 minutes at 25°C. Thereafter, Ehrlich's reagent (80μl) was added and plates were incubated in a shaking water bath for 20 minutes at 60°C. The extinction was read at 570nm.

Analysis of nitrite and nitrate

Nitrite and nitrate levels, both stable end products of nitric oxide, were measured spectrophotometrically in filtered (10kDa Biomax-Ultrafilters, Millipore, Bedford, Massachusetts, US) wound fluid as described above Schaffer et al., 1997a, 2002). In cell culture supernatants, as mentioned before, nitrite only was tested as an index of nitric-oxide synthesis.

Statistical analysis

All data are reported as means ± standard error of the mean (SEM). Statistical analysis was performed by applying *t*-test and ANOVA followed by Scheffé's test using the StatView II statistical package (Abacus Concepts, Berkeley, California). Statistical significance was set at $p<0.05$.

Results

Insulin treatment rendered diabetic BioBreeding rats normoglycaemic (day of wounding: 105 ± 11mg/dl; day 10: 99 ± 8mg/dl). Their blood glucose levels, measured daily in blood obtained from the tail vein, were not significantly different to those of the control animals (day of wounding: 95 ± 8mg/dl; day 10: 93 ± 8mg/dl, $p=0.09$ and $p=0.21$ respectively). Hyperglycaemic diabetic animals (who did not receive insulin treatment) exhibited significantly elevated blood glucose levels (day of wounding: 268 ± 23mg/dl; day 10: 255 ± 21mg/dl) when compared with the controls and normoglycaemic diabetic animals at all time points ($p<0.001$).

The wounding procedure was well tolerated by all animals in the study.

Post-wounding, the controls and normoglycaemic diabetic rats gained weight equally (control: $19 \pm 2\%$; normoglycaemic rats: $17 \pm 2\%$). In contrast, the hyperglycaemic diabetic animals did not gain weight post-wounding ($-0.4 \pm 3\%$). This was statistically significant different to the other two groups ($p<0.01$).

Plasma levels of total protein and albumin were similar in the normoglycaemic diabetic animals and the controls. However, the hyperglycaemic diabetic rats had decreased protein and albumin levels in plasma at 10 days post-wounding (*Table 1*).

In both the hyperglycaemic and normoglycaemic diabetic animals, wound collagen deposition and wound-breaking strength were significantly reduced ($p<0.01$) (*Figure 1*). There were no wound infections as assessed clinically and by testing wound fluid for sterility.

Impaired healing in the hyperglycaemic and normoglycaemic diabetic rats was paralleled by decreased wound-fluid nitrite and nitrate concentrations ($p<0.001$; *Figure 2*).

Wound-fluid protein concentrations decreased in the hyperglycaemic

Table 1. Total plasma protein and albumin levels, number of infiltrating cells per sponge and cell viability 10 days post-wounding

Group	Protein (g/dl)	Albumin (g/dl)	No of cells/ sponge	Cell viability
Control	4.98 ± 0.04	2.65 ± 0.04	3.4 ± 0.5x10⁶	61 ± 6
Normoglycaemic rats (diabetes plus insulin)	5.01 ± 0.05	2.60 ± 0.04	3.6 ± 0.6x10⁶	57 ± 7
Hyperglycaemic rates (diabetes)	4.29 ± 0.04*	2.32 ± 0.05*	2.5 ± 0.6 x 10⁶	56 ± 6

n = 10 rats in each group
*p<0.05 versus control and normoglycaemic rats
Results are presented as means ± standard error of the mean

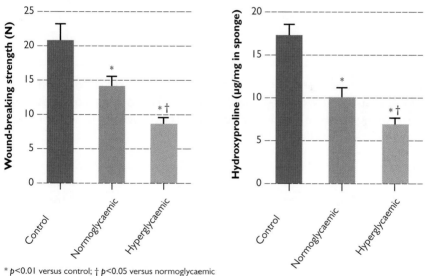

* *p*<0.01 versus control; † *p*<0.05 versus normoglycaemic
N = Newtons; normoglycaemic = diabetes plus insulin; hyperglycaemic = diabetes

Figure 1. Wound-breaking strength and wound collagen deposition at 10 days post-wounding.

diabetic animals (control: 50.4 ± 3.1mg/ml, normoglycaemic rats: 48.8 ± 2.9mg/ml, hyperglycaemic rats: 39.2 ± 2.6mg/ml; *p*<0.01).

The inflammatory response, measured as the number of infiltrating cells per sponge, was reduced in the hyperglycaemic diabetic rats (*Table 1*).

Systemic treatment with molsidomine was well tolerated by all animals. Molsidomine (4mg/kg/day) partially reversed wound nitrite and nitrate levels (*p*<0.01; *Table 2*). It also partially restored decreased wound

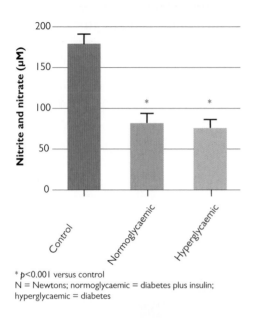

* p<0.001 versus control
N = Newtons; normoglycaemic = diabetes plus insulin;
hyperglycaemic = diabetes

Figure 2. Nitrite and nitrate concentrations in wound fluid at 10 days post-wounding.

Table 2. Effect of systemic treatment with a nitric oxide donor (molsidomine) on wound-breaking strength, sponge collages deposition (hydroxyproline) and nitrite plus nitrate levels in wound fluid 10 days post-wounding

Group	Wound-breaking strength (Newton)	Hydroxyproline (μg/mg sponge)	Nitrite plus nitrate in wound fluid (μM)
Control plus vehicle	20.4 ± 2.3	18.1 ± 2.5	168 ± 13
Normoglycaemic plus vehicle	12.3 ± 1.2*	9.6 ± 0.8*	74 ± 8*
Hyperglycaemic plus vehicle	7.4 ± 0.8*	6.3 ± 0.5*	69 ± 8*
Normoglycaeic plus molsidomine	18.7 ± 2.0[†]	16.9 ± 1.8[†]	102 ± 11[†+]
Hyperglycaemic plus molsidomine	14.1 ± 0.9*[§]	11.2 ± 0.9*[§]	92 ± 10*[§]

n = 10 rats in each group
Molsidomine dosage was 4mg/kg/day
* *p<0.01 versus control versus vehicle*
† *p<0.01 versus normoglycaemic plus vehicle*
+ *p<0.05 versus control plus vehicle*
§ *p<0.05 versus hyperglycaemic plus vehicle*
Results are presented as means ± standards error of the mean

Table 3. Spontaneous release of nitrite (index of nitric-oxide synthesis) and hydroxyproline (index of collagen production) by first-passage fibroblasts harvested 10 days post-wounding

Group	Nitrite (nmol/24h/5x10⁵ cells)	Hydroxyproline (ng/24h/5x10⁵ cells)
Control	9.2 ± 1.4	718 ± 32
Normoglycaemic rats (diabetes plus insulin)	$1.1 \pm 0.2*$	$273 \pm 26*$
Hyperglycaemic rats (diabetes)	$1.0 \pm 0.2*$	$261 \pm 24*$

n = 10 rats in each group
* p<0.001 versus control
Results are presented as means ± standard error of the mean

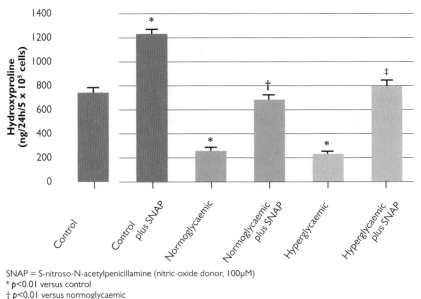

SNAP = S-nitroso-N-acetylpenicillamine (nitric-oxide donor, 100μM)
* *p*<0.01 versus control
† *p*<0.01 versus normoglycaemic
‡ *p*<0.01 versus hyperglycaemic

Figure 3. Release of hydroxyproline by first-passage fibroblasts harvested 10 days post-wounding in response to normal culture media and culture media plus SNAP.

collagen deposition and wound mechanical strength in the hyperglycaemic diabetic animals.

In the normoglycaemic diabetic animals it reversed compromised healing close to the control levels (*p*<0.01; *Table 2*).

Ex vivo, fibroblasts isolated from 10-day-old wounds of the control animals spontaneously synthesised large amounts of nitric oxide. Nitric-oxide synthesis by wound fibroblasts obtained from hyperglycaemic and normoglycaemic diabetic rats was significantly reduced ($p<0.001$; *Table 3*). This was paralleled by a decreased *ex vivo* collagen synthesis by wound fibroblasts from normoglycaemic and hyperglycaemic diabetic rats ($p<0.01$, *Figure 3*).

In vitro nitric-oxide donor treatment increased collagen production in fibroblasts from control animals to supranormal levels. In fibroblasts derived from hyperglycaemic and normoglycaemic diabetic animals, exogenous nitric oxide reversed *ex vivo* collagen synthesis similar to control levels (*Figure 3*).

Discussion

These results show that wound healing was impaired in hyperglycaemic (non-insulin treated) and normoglycaemic (insulin-treated) diabetic rats.

Impaired healing was reflected by diminished wound nitric-oxide production and decreased synthesis of nitric oxide and collagen by wound-derived fibroblasts. However, exogenous nitric oxide was able to reverse impaired healing and diminished fibroblast activity.

A hyperglycaemic state of diabetes has been shown to be related to impaired healing and diminished wound nitric-oxide synthesis (Schaffer et al., 1997a; Wetzler et al., 2000; Witte et al., 2002a, b). Little is known, however, about the role of nitric oxide in wound repair in a model of normoglycaemic type I diabetes. It is still unclear whether the alterations observed in diabetic wound repair relate to hyperglycaemia or modified cellular activity in normo-glycaemic diabetic disease.

In keeping with our findings, hyperglycaemic diabetic animals have exhibited a catabolic state (Schaffer et al., 1997a). Furthermore, nutritional parameters, including albumin and total protein in plasma and wound fluid, are reduced. Weight loss associated with poor nutritional food intake and lack of individual nutrients, even of a short duration, impairs healing (Greenhalgh and Gamelli, 1987; Yue et al., 1987). Similarly, delayed healing following acute protein-calorie malnutrition is associated with decreased wound nitric-oxide production (Schaffer et al., 1997c).

It is thus conceivable that, at least in part, some of the effects investigated in hyperglycaemic diabetic wound healing are not due to specific diabetic alterations but may be caused by malnutrition (Yue et al., 1987).

In our experiments normoglycaemic diabetic rats and the controls gained weight equally throughout the study. Also, albumin and protein blood levels and wound-fluid protein concentrations were similar in the normoglycaemic rats and controls, suggesting that malnutrition did not affect healing outcomes in the insulin-treated animals.

The inflammatory response, measured as the number of viable infiltrating cells per sponge, was not significantly different between the normoglycaemic diabetic animals and the controls. In contrast, the hyperglycaemic diabetic animals exhibited a decreased number of wound-infiltrating cells. This is in keeping with another study that investigated the role of hyperglycaemia on wound healing (Witte et al., 2002a).

Again, hyperglycaemia accompanied by a significant weight loss seems to mimic a different state of wound immune function when compared with normoglycaemia. In hyperglycaemia, a decreased total number of wound-infiltrating cells, rather than decreased cellular activity, may be responsible for impaired healing.

In our experiments insulin-treated diabetic animals were made normoglycaemic for one week before wounding. It remains unclear whether a longer preoperative period of normoglycaemia would affect the level of collagen and nitric-oxide synthesis. The insulin-treated animals, however, were not found to be different to the non-diabetic controls with respect to weight gain, plasma and wound-fluid protein levels, and the inflammatory response in the wound. These findings indicate that normogylcaemic diabetic rats have a steady metabolic state. The ensuing effect on the wound environment, in turn, modulates the phenotype of fibroblasts present in the wound (Regan et al., 1991; Schaffer et al., 1997d).

Furthermore, in our *in vitro* experiments the addition of exogenous nitric oxide for only 24 hours completely restored decreased fibroblast activity in the diabetic animals, suggesting that a change in the wound environment (insulin therapy or nitric oxide treatment) may affect the fibroblast phenotype *in vivo* within hours.

Nitric oxide has been shown to play a significant role in wound repair (Schaffer et al., 1996 ; Yamasaki et al., 1998).Inhibition of wound nitric-oxide synthesis decreases wound mechanical strength and collagen deposition. In turn, supplementation of nitric oxide partially restores impaired healing, suggesting that it plays a key role in the complex cascade of cellular and biochemical events that occur after injury to restore host integrity.

On the cellular level, nitric oxide is synthesised in the wound mainly by macrophages and fibroblasts (Schaffer et al., 1997b). Due to their ultimate role in collagen synthesis, fibroblasts are of key interest during the proliferation phase of healing. Fibroblast activity to synthesise collagen is regulated by nitric oxide in an autocrine and paracrine fashion (Schaffer et al., 1997b). A posttranscriptional regulatory mechanism has to be postulated since nitric oxide does not affect collagen gene transcription in fibroblasts (Witte et al., 2000).

It appears that the activity of wound-derived fibroblasts to synthesise nitric oxide and collagen is decreased in normoglycaemic diabetic rats. Exogenous supplementation of nitric oxide restores wound-repair mechanisms. This is reflected in increased wound fibroblast collagen synthesis.

From our results, however, we cannot conclude whether the *in vivo* application of the nitric-oxide donor directly stimulated fibroblasts to synthesise more collagen or whether this is secondary to other stimulatory mediators, such as TGF-beta, released by different wound cells in response to the exogenous nitric oxide.

Our *in vitro* results, however, suggest that, at least in part, the *in vivo* effects observed in nitric-oxide treated wounds are directly correlated to a stimulatory effect on wound fibroblasts. Collagen synthesis in wound-derived fibroblasts from control animals is not maximal since the addition of exogenous nitric oxide further stimulated fibroblast activity.

The addition of nitric oxide at high concentrations has been found to inhibit hepatocyte and smooth muscle protein synthesis (Curran et al., 1991; Kolpakov et al., 1995). Those experiments have shown that inhibition of protein synthesis requires high nitric-oxide concentrations and may be due to cell toxicity in some cases.

In non-diabetic dermal fibroblasts, the addition of nitric-oxide donors in low concentrations (50–100μM) has been shown to stimulate collagen synthesis, but higher doses decreased total protein and collagen production (Witte et al., 1996).

The stimulatory effect of nitric oxide on collagen synthesis appears to be a very specific and important regulator of a critical fibroblast function during the repair process, particularly since the level of total protein synthesis seems to be affected (Schaffer et al., 1997b).

Impaired healing in diabetes is not limited to diminished nitric-oxide metabolism. All phases of the complex healing cascade, including inflammation, proliferation and matrix formation, are affected. Reduced chemotaxis, phagocytosis, bacterial killing and antioxidant levels during the early phase of healing have been reported in hyperglycaemic diabetes (Sima et al.,1988; Marhoffer et al., 1992; Mohan and Das, 1998).Growth factor depletion, decreased cell proliferation, diminished fibroblast-mediated collagen matrix contraction and collagen synthesis, and upregulation of apoptosis characterise the later phase of diabetic healing (Bitar and Labbad, 1996; Darby et al., 1997; Witte et al., 2002a).

Therapeutically, local administration of growth factors has been tested, but clinical results have been mostly disappointing (Albertson et al., 1993; Wieman et al., 1998; Petrova and Edmonds, 2006). Insulin treatment restores some of the effects observed in hyperglycaemic diabetes, but may not reverse all deficits of diabetic healing. Exogenous nitric oxide has shown some promising results in delayed-healing diabetic wounds (Witte et al., 2002a; Weller and Finnen, 2006). According to our results, this may not only be true for well-known states of hyperglycaemia but may also count for the metabolic steady state of normoglycaemia.

Conclusion

The results of this study demonstrated that collagen deposition was reduced in wounds in both the normoglycaemic and hyperglycaemic diabetic rats. Significantly, the rate of healing was greater in the normoglycaemic diabetic rats, who did not experience weight loss.

Exogenous nitric oxide improved wound repair in both groups, but the rate of healing was better in the normoglycaemic diabetic rats.

Malnutrition affects wound healing. The hyperglycaemic diabetic rats lost weight when compared with the normogylcaemic rats and the controls. Therefore, the exact mechanism that affects wound healing in poorly controlled diabetes has yet to be identified.

It is still not clear how much exogenous nitric oxide is needed to promote wound healing. In fact, because of its toxic effects, too much nitric oxide may be deleterious. Further research is therefore needed to confirm this.

References

Albertson S, Hummel RP, Breeden M, Greenhalgh DG (1993) PDGF und FGF reverse the healing impairment in protein-malnourished diabetic mice. *Surg* **114**: 368–72

Bitar MS, Labbad ZN (1996) TGF-beta and IGF-I in relation to diabetes-induced impairment of wound healing. *J Surg Res* **61**: 113–19

Creemers LB, Jansen DC, van Veen-Reurings A (1997) Microassay for assessment of low levels of hydroxyproline. **Bio Techniques 22**: 656–61

Curran RD, Ferrari FK, Kispert PH et al. (1991) Nitric oxide and nitric oxide-generating compounds inhibit hepatocyte protein synthesis. *FASEB J* 5: 2085–92

Darby IA, Bisucci T, Hewitson TD, MacLellan DG (1997) Apoptosis is increased in a model of diabetes-impaired wound healing in genetically diabetic mice. J Biochem Cell Biol **29**: 191–200

Falanga V (2005) Wound healing and its impairment of the diabetic foot. *Lancet* **366**: 1736–43

Follak N, Kloting L, Wolf E, Merk H (2004) Delayed remodeling in the early period of fracture healing in spontaneously diabetic BB/OK rats depending on the diabetic metabolic state. *Histol Histopathol* **19**: 473–86

Goodson WH, Hunt TK (1977) Studies of wound healing in experimental diabetes. *J Surg Res* **22**: 221–7

Greenhalgh DG, Gamelli RL (1987) Is impaired wound healing caused by infection or nutritional depletion? *Surgery* **102**: 306–12

Kolpakov V, Gordon D, Kulik TJ (1995) Nitric oxide-generating compounds inhibit total protein and collagen synthesis in cultured vascular smooth muscle cells. *Circ Res* 76: 305–9

Marhoffer W, Stein M, Maeser E, Ferderlin K (1992) Impairment of polymorphonuclear leukocyte function and metabolic control of diabetes. *Diabetes Care* **15**: 256–60

Mohan IK, Das UN (1998) Effect of arginine-NO system on chemical induced diabetes mellitus. *Free Radic Biol Med* **25**: 757–65

Petrova N, Edmonds M (2006) Emerging drugs for diabetic foot ulcers. *Expert Opin Drugs* **11**: 709–24

Regan MC, Kirk SJ, Wasserkrzg HL, Barbul A (1991) The wound environment as a regulator of fibroblast phenotype. *J Surg Res* **50**: 442–8

Schäffer M, Efron PA, Thornton FJ et al. (1997b) Nitric oxide, an autokrine regulator of wound fibroblast synthetic function. *J Immunol* **158**: 2375–81

Schäffer M, Tantry U, Ahrendt G et al. (1997c) Acute protein-calorie malnutrition impairs wound healing: a possible role of decreased wound nitric oxide synthesis. *J Am Coll Surg* **184**: 37–43

Schäffer M, Tantry U, Ahrendt G et al. (1997d) Stimulation of fibroblast proliferation and matrix contraction by wound fluid. *Int J Biochem Cell Biol* **29**: 231–9

Schäffer M, Tantry U, Efron PA et al. (1997a) Diabetes-impaired healing and reduced wound nitric oxide synthesis: a possible pathophysiologic correlation. *Surg* **121**: 513–19

Schäffer M, Weimer W, Wider S et al. (2002) Differential expression of inflammatory mediators in radiation-impaired wound healing. *J Surg Res* **107**: 93–100

Yamasaki K, Edington HDJ, McClosky C et al. (1998) Reversal of impaired wound repair in iNOS–deficient mice by topical adenoviral-mediated iNOS gene transfer. *J Clin Invest* **101**: 967–71

Schäffer M, Tantry U, Gross SS et al. (1996) Nitric oxide regulates wound healing. *J Surg Res* **63**: 237–40

Sima AA, O'Neill SJ, Naimark D et al. (1988) Bacterial phagocytosis and intracellular killing by alveolar macrophages in BB rats. *Diabetes* **37**: 544–9

Tyndall WA, Beam HA, Zarro C et al. (2003) Decreased platelet derived growth factor expression during fracture healing in diabetic animals. *Clin Orthop Relat Res* **408**: 319–30

Weller R, Finnen MJ (2006) The effects of topical treatment with acidified nitrite on wound healing in normal and diabetic mice. *Nitric Oxide* **15**: 395–439

Wetzler C, Kampfer H, Stallmeyer B et al. (2000) Large and sustained induction of chemokines during impaired wound healing in the genetically diabetic mouse: prolonged persistence of neutrophils and macrophages during the late phase of repair. *J Invest Dermatol* **115**: 245–53

Wieman TJ, Smiell JM, Su Y (1998) Efficacy and safety of a topical gel formulation of recombinant human platelet-derived growth factor-BB (becaplermin) in patients with chronic neuropathic diabetic ulcers:a phase III randomized placebo-controlled double-blind study. *Diabetes Care* **21**: 822–9

Witte MB, Kiyama T, Barbul A (2002a) Nitric oxide enhances experimental wound healing in diabetes. *Br J Surg* **89**: 1594–601

Witte MB, Schäffer MR, Barbul A (1996) Phenotypic induction of nitric oxide is critical for synthetic function in wound fibroblasts. *Surg Forum* **47**: 703–5

Witte MB, Thornton FJ, Efron DT, Barbul A (2000) Enhancement of fibroblast collagen synthesis by nitric oxide. *Nitric Oxide* **4**: 572–82

Witte MB, Thornton FJ, Tantry U, Barbul A (2002b) L-arginine supplementation enhances diabetic wound healing: involvement of the nitric oxide synthase and arginase pathways. *Metabolism* **51:** 1269–73

Woessner J (1961) The determination of hydroxyproline in tissue and protein samples containing small proportions of this amino acid. *Arch Biochem Biophys* **93**: 440–7

Yang Y, Santamaria P (2006) Lessons on autoimmune diabetes from animal models. *Clin Sci (London)* **110**: 627–39

Yue DK, McLennan S, Marish M et al. (1987) Effects of experimental diabetes, uremia, and malnutrition on wound healing. *Diabetes* **36**: 295–9

An overview of the two widely accepted, but contradictory, theories on wound contraction

S Pellard

Wound contraction is a final feature of the proliferation phase, and is defined as the mechanism by which the edges of an open wound are drawn together as a result of forces within the wound (Van Winkle, 1967).

Contraction begins four to five days after wounding, at an average rate of 0.6 to 0.75mm/day, and is influenced by the wound shape and size, whether the wound is dressed or exposed, the age of the individual, the type of animal wounded and the anatomical location of the wound (Van Winkle, 1967).

Influences on wound contraction

Wound size and shape

Early experiments (Spain and Loeb, 1915; Carrel and Hartmann, 1916) revealed that:

- The rate of contraction is greater at the beginning than at the end of the repair period
- Contraction is dependent on the area rather than the age of the wound
- The larger the wound, the greater the rate of contraction.

Carrel and Hartmann (1916) studied wounds in humans, cats and guinea pigs. All the wounds were dressed, which may have interfered with healing, although it should be noted that the study was undertaken before the need for a moist wound healing environment was identified. The human wounds had different anatomical sites and mechanisms of injury, and were of varying durations, but this was not accounted for in the study.

The wound shape also influences the rate of contraction. Circular wounds contract at a slower rate than rectangular wounds (Billingham and Russell, 1956). In the latter, the corners move more slowly than the central points of the linear edges (Van Winkle, 1967).

Age of the wound

In vivo experiments have shown that wounds in the young contract faster than those in adults, and there is a gradual decline in the speed of contraction during adult life (Billingham and Russell, 1956).

Animal and human wounds

Few recent studies have been undertaken in human models (Berry et al., 1998). Wound contraction is slower in humans than in animals (Berry et al., 1998), and most animals have large areas of loose skin, so wound closure occurs with little scarring or loss of function.

In humans, the skin is more firmly attached to underlying tissues, so the consequences of contraction range from a cosmetic scar to loss of joint movement or body deformation (Billingham and Medawar, 1955).

The wound site

Extremity wounds exposed to air show minimal contraction when compared with sacrococcygeal wounds, which heal predominantly by contraction: Berry et al. (1998) demonstrated that contraction contributed to 88% of sacrococcygeal wound closure, whereas scar deposition was only 12%.

Wounds on Langer's lines have less granulation tissue because contraction narrows the cavity and occurs at right angles to the lines of skin tension. Surgical wounds should therefore be planned in relation to these (Watts, 1960).

Wound contraction theories

Two widely accepted but contradictory theories have been proposed for wound contraction:

- Cell contraction theory (Gabbiani et al., 1971)
- Cell traction theory (Ehrlich and Rajaratnam, 1990).

Cell contraction theory

This proposes that myofibroblasts situated within granulation tissue contract (Gabbiani et al., 1971). The synchronised cellular contraction pulls collagen fibrils towards the body of the myofibroblast, holding the fibrils until their position is stabilised (Rudolph, 1980; Skalli and Gabbiani, 1988). This coordinated gathering of collagen fibres towards the body of the myofibroblast leads to the shrinkage of granulation tissue. As the extracellular matrix is continuous with the undamaged edge of the wound, this shrinkage of the granulation tissue pulls the wound margin and leads to wound contraction.

The myofibroblast was identified in 1971. It was defined as a cell with the characteristics of smooth muscle cells and fibroblasts, including:

- Abundant rough endoplasmic reticulum
- Intercellular junctions (desmosomes, gap junctions and fibronexus)
- Actin microfilament bundles attached to the cell membrane, parallel to the long axis of the cell
- Multilobulated (numerous deep folds) and indented nuclei during contraction (Gabbiani et al., 1971).

It has been postulated that myofibroblasts are derived from at least three mesenchymal cells including fibroblasts, smooth muscle cells and pericytes, all of which express alpha-smooth muscle actin (αSMA), smooth muscle myosin and desmin (Schmitt-Graff et al., 1994). Desmin is a marker of general muscular differentiation; smooth muscle myosin is a specific marker of smooth muscle differentiation, but disappears *in vivo*; αSMA, which is present in all smooth muscle cells, is the most reliable marker of smooth muscle origin, suggesting that myofibroblasts temporarily acquire some smooth muscle features to aid contraction (Darby et al., 1990). Desmouliere et al. (2005) suggested that myofibroblasts are derived from fibroblasts, and that the transition starts with the appearance of the protomyofibroblast.

Myofibroblasts have been further divided into five phenotypes, according to variations in cytoskeletal protein expression. However, this causes difficulties when comparing research data as definitions of myofibroblasts vary between authors, so cell populations of myofibroblasts may not be comparable. Cultured fibroblasts cause problems because αSMA expression depends on culture conditions and does not correlate with expression *in vivo* (Nedelec et al., 2000).

When wound contraction ceases and the wound is fully epithelialised, myofibroblasts containing αSMA disappear, probably by apoptosis, and the scar becomes less cellular (Desmouliere, 1995). The signals leading to this disappearance are still unknown.

Cell traction theory

The cell traction theory suggests that fibroblasts exert uncoordinated 'traction forces' on the extracellular matrix fibres to which they are attached, allowing a closer approximation of matrix fibrils. *In vitro* studies, using cells from different aged parts of chicken embryos, show that the traction force of fibroblasts is strong enough to distort collagen gels and form patterns of tension, compression and alignment, similar to wrinkling patterns previously observed on silicone rubber. The wrinkling is believed to represent the gathering of collagen fibres during their remodelling by fibroblasts (Harris et al, 1981; Stopak and Harris, 1982).

Ehrlich (1988) demonstrated *in vitro* the contraction capacity of fibroblast collagen matrices. He rejected the idea that myofibroblasts are responsible for wound contraction as he found no difference in contraction between lattices enriched or deficient in them (Ehrlich, 1988).

McGrath and Hundahl's (1982) pig study quantified myofibroblasts in granulation tissue by immunoperoxidase labelling. They studied myofibroblast distribution in a granulating wound and found that it correlated to the rate of wound contraction over time. Increased numbers of myofibroblasts were also seen near the inflammatory foci in the granulation tissue, which was statistically significant, and contraction rates did not alter in wounds with different tension loads. Although this study supports the theory that the myofibroblast is responsible for wound contraction, it did state that the contractile fibroblast, not the myofibroblast, predates the onset of wound contraction. Darby et al. (1990) supported this finding. These results have not been reproduced in humans. However, Majno et al. (1997), in a rat study, could not identify any myofibroblast cells when wound contraction was 50% complete.

In vitro experiments (Erhlich, 1988; Ehrlich and Rajaratnam, 1990) with contracting fibroblast-populated collagen lattices (FPCL), a dermal equivalent that is able to contract over time and is enriched or deficient in myofibroblasts, showed that contraction was slower in areas of abundant myofibroblasts. Contraction was slower at the periphery, where there are more intercellular connections than in the central areas of the lattice. However, FPCL contraction occurs rapidly, and is difficult to compare to *in vivo* wound contraction, which is a steady active process occurring over a relatively long time period.

Postlethwaite et al. (1987) suggested that fibroblasts that are rich in F-actin bundles generate the force of contraction. Stimuli such as fibronectin, platelet-derived growth factor (PDGF) or transforming growth factor-beta (TGF-β) draw fibroblasts into the wound, which then undergo a phenotypic change. They synthesise type I collagen, fibronectin and other ground substance proteins, perhaps in response to TGF-β (Sporn et al., 1987). Initially, fibronectin is confined to the fibroblast surface, but within a few days linkages occur between cells, and fibroblasts express fibronectin receptors from bundles of F-actin along the axis of their peripheral cytoplasm. They become elongated and aligned with each other and the fibronectin/collagen matrix, and wound contraction then occurs.

It has been suggested that the newly formed extracellular matrix is linked together and to the surrounding tissue, and that contraction occurs as tension on the matrix draws the surrounding tissue inward (Welch et al., 1990). Cellular-generated forces reorganise collagen through the mechanical translocation of the collagen fibrils, where fine collagen fibrils become thicker and longer fibres (Berry et al., 1998).

Attempts have been made to combine these two contradictory theories of wound contraction, suggesting that myofibroblast differentiation may be stimulated by the locomotion of fibroblasts, generating mechanical contractile forces *in vivo* (Grinnell, 1994).

Conclusion

Wound contraction appears to be mediated by cells from the fibroblast lineage, and both fibroblast and myofibroblast cells appear to interact with the extracellular matrix to achieve contraction. Many studies support the cell contraction theory (McGrath and Hundahl, 1982; Darby et al., 1990; Schmitt-Graff et al., 1994; Desmouliere, 1995) and the cell traction theory

(Harris et al., 1981; Ehrlich, 1988; Ehrlich and Rajaratnam, 1990), but experimental proof of the exact mechanism of contraction varies greatly between studies. The fact that most were *in vitro* studies using different culture mediums and models is the most likely cause of the conflicting results. Tejero-Trujeque (2001) suggested that conflicting results in understanding the mechanism of wound contraction are due to the lack of an *in vitro* true skin equivalent.

More research is needed to identify the exact mechanism of wound contraction. While *in vitro* studies allow far greater control of the experimental system and easier measurements, they are unable to fully mimic the true wound environment and tend to examine one specific cell type. Norman (2004) suggested that further human and animal studies are required to establish all the cell interactions

References

Berry DP, Harding KG, Stanton MR et al. (1988) Human wound contraction: collagen organization, fibroblasts and myofibroblasts. *Plastic Reconstr Surg* **102**(1): 124–31

Billingham RE, Medawar PB (1955) Contracture and intussusceptive growth in healing of extensive wounds in mammalian skin. *J Anat* **89**(1): 114–23

Billingham RE, Russell PS (1956) Studies on wound healing, with special reference to the phenomenon of contracture in experimental wounds in rabbits' skin. *Annal Surg* **144**: 6, 961–81

Carrel A, Hartmann A (1916) Cicatrisation of wounds. *J Exp Med* **24**: 429–50

Darby I, Skalli O, Gabbiani G (1990) Alpha-smooth muscle actin is transiently expressed by myofibroblasts during experimental wound healing. *Laboratory Investigations* **63**(1): 21–9

Desmouliere A (1995) Factors influencing myofibroblast differentiation during wound healing and fibrosis. *Cell Biol Int* **19**(5): 471–6

Desmouliere A, Chaponnier C, Gabbiani G (2005) Tissue repair, contraction, and the myofibroblast. Wound Repair Regen **13**(1): 7–12

Ehrlich HP (1988) Wound closure: evidence of cooperation between fibroblasts and collagen matrix. *Eye* **2**(pt 2): 149–57

Ehrlich HP, Rajaratnam JBM (1990) Cell locomotion forces versus cell contraction forces for collagen lattice contraction: an in vitro model of wound contraction. *Tissue Cell* **22**(4): 407–17

Gabbiani G, Ryan GB, Majno G (1971) Presence of modified fibroblasts in granulation tissue and their possible role in wound contraction. *Experimentia* **27**(5): 549–50

Grinnell F (1994) Fibroblasts, myofibroblasts and wound contraction. *J Cell Biol* **124**(4): 401–4

Harris AK, Stopak D, Wild P (1981) Fibroblast traction as a mechanism for collagen morphogenesis. *Nature* **290**: 249–51

Majno G, Gabbiani G, Hirschel BJ et al. (1997) Contraction of granulation tissue in vitro: similarity to smooth muscle. *Science* **173**: 548–50

McGrath MH, Hundahl SA (1982) The spatial and temporal quantification of myofibroblasts. *Plast Reconstr Surg* **69**(6): 975–85

Nedelec B, Ghahary A, Scott PG, Tredget EE (2000) Control of wound contraction: basic and clinical features. *Hand Clin* **16**(2): 289–302

Norman D (2004) An exploration of two opposing theories of wound contraction. *J Wound Care* **13**(4): 138–40 Postlethwaite AE, Keski-Oja J, Moses HL, Kang AH (1987) Stimulation of the chemotactic migration of human fibroblasts by transforming growth factor-beta. *J Exp Med* **165**(1): 251–6

Postlethwaite AE, Keski-Oja J, Moses HL, Kang AH (1987) Stimulation of the chemotactic migration of human fibroblasts by transforming growth factor-beta. *J Exp Med* **165**(1): 251–6

Rudolph R (1980) Contraction and the control of contraction. *World J Surg* **4**: 279–87

Schmitt-Graff A, Desmouliere A, Gabbiani G (1994) Heterogeneity of myofibroblast phenotypic features: an example of fibroblastic cell plasticity. *Virchows Archiv* **425**(1): 3–24

Skalli O, Gabbiani G (1988) The biology of the myofibroblast relationship to wound contraction and fibrocontractive diseases. In: Clark RAF, Henson PM (eds) *Molecular and Cellular Biology of Wound Repair*. Plenum

Spain KC, Loeb L (1915) A quantitative analysis of the influence of the size of the defect on wound healing in the skin of the guinea pig. *J Exp Med* **23**: 107–22

Sporn MB, Roberts AB, Wakefield LM, de Crombrugghe B (1987) Some recent advances in the chemistry and biology of transforming growth factor-beta. *J Cell Biol* **105**(3): 1039–45

Stopak D, Harris AK (1982) Connective tissue morphogenesis by fibroblast traction: I. Tissue culture observations. *Dev Biol* **90**(2): 383–98

Tejero-Trujeque R (2001) How do fibroblasts interact with the extracellular matrix in wound contraction? *J Wound Care* **10**(6): 237–42

Van Winkle W Jr (1967) Wound contraction. *Surg Gynaecol Obstet* **125**(1): 131–42

Watts GT (1960) Wound shape and tissue tension in healing. *Br J Surg* **47**: 555–61

Welch MP, Odland GF, Clark RAF (1990) Temporal relationships of F-actin bundle formation, collagen and fibronectin matrix assembly, and fibronectin receptor expression to wound contraction. *J Cell Biol* **110**(1): 133–45

A study of biofilm-based wound management in subjects with critical limb ischaemia

R D Wolcott and D D Rhoads

There are many barriers to wound healing, and wound-care providers identify and manage a myriad of wound barriers every day. For example, each patient with a wound is evaluated each visit for poor perfusion, acute infection, poor nutrition, repetitive pressure, unmanaged medical disease, and so on. Unfortunately, even when these barriers are managed well, patient outcomes do not seem to be significantly improved (McIsaac, 2005; Akopian et al., 2006).

Additionally, some nagging questions about chronic wounds exist. For example, why does a chronic wound often persist longer than a neighbouring acute wound that arises during the course of therapy (*Figure 1*)? Why does an acute traumatic wound that is closed with sutures after it has been present for more than eight hours run a greater risk of wound dehiscence than if it were closed after a shorter period of time (Reynolds and Cole, 2006)? In the traumatic wound, current planktonic (single cell) concepts suggest that more bacteria have accumulated in the older wound, which has led to colonisation. Fortunately, planktonic bacteria are sensitive to antibiotics and biocides, so a prolonged surgical scrub should eliminate the increased bacteria. However, even if a more aggressive surgical scrub is used on the wound, the results from primary closure after eight hours remain poor. What is the explanation for the poor healing of chronic wounds?

The possible role of biofilm in preventing chronic wound healing

Bacterial biofilms may be the unrecognised but important barrier that impairs the healing of chronic wounds (*Table 1*). The concept of biofilm

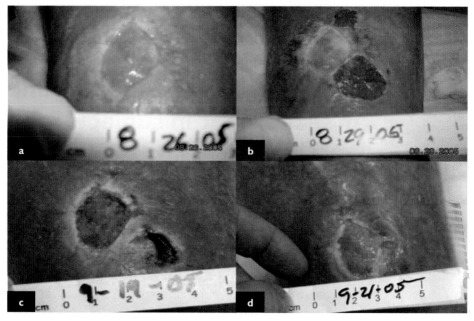

Figure 1. The initial chronic wound demonstrates a thick film on its surface (a). Three days later, the film is still visible on the initial wound, but a new satellite wound shows no significant film (b). Biofilm-based wound-care strategies were immediately used on the fresh satellite wound, and it quickly healed within two weeks (c). Presumably, a biofilm was not allowed to establish on the satellite wound because of immediate management. However, the established wound persisted for three additional weeks after the acute wound healed. The presence or absence of wound biofilm is the best explanation for this observed dichotomy in healing (d).

is not well known in medicine (Costerton et al., 1999), and it is only beginning to be understood in the basic scientific community. Biofilm is created when a single-cell planktonic bacterium adheres to the surface of the wound by attaching to the exposed extracellular matrix proteins. The bacteria can rapidly begin expressing extracellular polymeric substance (EPS) and up to 800 new proteins to form a microcolony within hours (Sauer et al., 2002). Within 10 hours, each single-cell planktonic bacterium has differentiated into a complex community with impressive multiple colony defences (Harrison-Balestra et al., 2003), including an increased resistance to antibiotics (Sauer et al., 2002), biocides, and human immunity (Costerton et al., 1999; Fux et al, 2005). Recent molecular studies have demonstrated that wound biofilms are polymicrobial communities containing more bacterial species than are revealed using routine clinical culture (James et al., 2007; Dowd et al., 2008a, b). It is plausible that this natural bacterial

Table 1. Planktonic versus biofilm explanation for clinical observations (Woolcott, 2007)

Observation	Planktonic concept	Biofilm concept
In vitro	Planktonic bacterium (seed) expresses proteins and structures for motility and attachment (flagella, fimbria). Its function is to spread the colony to a different location	Biofilm (vegetation) is a complex colony of bacteria that can express different proteins (variable phenotype) to fulfil different roles to help the community survive. Biofilm is stationary, protecting its location with multiple defences
In vivo	Planktonic bacteria are susceptible to antibiotics, biocides and the immune system	Biofilms are resistant to antibiotics and biocides. Once biofilm is established it cannot be eradicated by the immune system
Acute wounds health in 2–4 weeks; chronic wounds in the same area heal in 4–6 months	Acute wounds have intact defences and destroy planktonic bacteria, not allowing biofilm formation	Some bacteria may evade host defences and establish a biofilm. Biofilm possesses defences against the host immune system and interferes with wound healing
Antibiotics are ineffective in chronic wounds but effective in acute wounds	Rapidly growing bacteria show a 4- to 5-log reduction in viability	The biofilm phenotypes quickly adapt and demonstrate only a grudging 1- to 2-log reduction, even at 50 to 1000 times the minimum inhibitory concentration (MIC)
Autograft or allograft fails on wounds	Planktonic cells are easily cleared by neutrophils, antibodies, and common wound bed preparations and so do not explain graft failure	Laying unprotected cells over biofilm adds a second surface and a food source. This leads to the rapid deterioration of the graft and increased exudate, inflammation and malodour
Negative wound cultures	Most clinical bacteria in planktonic phenotype are easily cultured	Wounds have bacteria on their surface yet can culture negative when a biofilm phenotype is present (ie, viable but not culturable)
Wounds 'stuck' in chronic inflammatory state	Planktonic bacteria are easily cleared by host inflammatory response and survive best if inflammation is avoided	Biofilms are impervious to the host inflammatory response and can even feed off the exudate produced by inflammation. Biofilms often promote inflammation

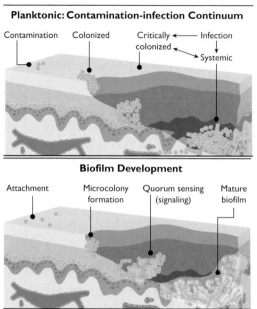

Planktonic: Contamination-infection Continuum

Figure 2. The first wound (top) represents a traditional model of infection. In this traditional paradigm, the bacteria progress from contaminants to colonisers to infectors. This traditional model focuses on the number of bacterial cells that can be cultured from a wound, and it may be a good picture of the agents that cause acute symptoms during an acute infection. However, we suggest that chronic wounds typically have an underlying infection that does not yield a flamboyant, acute host response but which delays host healing.

The second wound (bottom) represents this chronic, underlying biofilm infection. These biofilms can develop from a small number of contaminating bacteria, which can attach to the wound, develop into microcolonies and mature into a robust biofilm community that interacts using chemical signalling. Mature biofilms often comprise many genotypically distinct constituents, and each genotype can produce cells with various phenotypes. This diversity and quantity of cells in a biofilm cannot be determined effectively using traditional culturing techniques, so more sensitive diagnostic tools are needed to better identify the organisms causing chronic biofilm infections.

development into a biofilm is a cause for impaired healing in cutaneous wounds (*Figure 2*) (Bjarnsholt et al., 2008).

The presence of biofilm on the surface of chronic wounds has been alluded to for several years (Kalani et al., 1999; Bellow et al., 2001; Serralta et al., 2001; Mertz, 2003; Welsh et al., 2003; Clutterbuck et al., 2007) and has recently been demonstrated (James et al., 2007). James evaluated the wound beds of 50 chronic wounds and 16 acute wounds using scanning electron microscopy (SEM) to determine the presence of biofilm (*Figure 3*) (James et al., 2007). Biopsies of the 50 chronic wounds showed that 60% of the wound beds demonstrated definite biofilm. Of the 16 acute wounds, only one showed a small patch of biofilm on the wound bed. The study concluded that chronic wounds showed evidence of biofilm significantly more often than acute wounds. These differences between the chronic wounds and acute wounds in the presence of biofilm can help explain their different treatment outcomes.

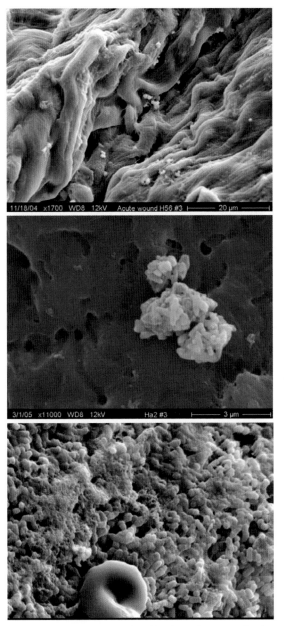

Figure 3. Acute wounds demonstrate biofilm less frequently than chronic wounds. A representative scanning electron micrograph of an acute wound shows the host's extracellular matrix with occasional bacterial clusters dotted across the landscape (a). In wounds, bacteria multiply to form microcolonies (b) that can develop into mature biofilms (c). Host defences and antibacterial agents have impaired effects on biofilm bacteria. (Electron micrographs courtesy of Ellen Swogger and Garth James, Center for Biofilm Engineering).

Treating biofilm infections

Biofilm-based infection management is very new to the medical community, yet the National Institutes of Health estimate up to 80% of human infectious disease is biofilm-based (National Institutes of Health, 1997; Costerton et al., 1999).

One of the most studied areas of human biofilm disease is oral biofilm. When a dental patient develops a biofilm disease (periodontal disease) the dentist recommends increased brushing, flossing, and ultrasonic removal of biofilm (plaque) to decrease the amount of biofilm that is causing the disease. In the moist environment of the mouth, a mature biofilm forms within 48 hours, requiring frequent debridement (brushing twice a day) (Leung et al., 2005). This aggressive debridement of the biofilm is used because it is known to improve patients' outcomes.

Frequent surgical debridement in wounds has also been found to lead to improved wound healing trajectories and improved total number of wounds healed (Apelqvist et al., 1993). The ischaemic wound bed is often cooler and drier than the mouth, so the ischaemic wound may be a less favourable environment for the growth of pathogenic bacteria in comparison to the oral cavity, which may explain why weekly (instead of daily) debridement is often of sufficient frequency to manage wounds complicated by critical limb ischaemia (CLI).

In addition to debridement, patients with certain types of biofilm disease are routinely treated with extensive courses of antibiotics. For example, in endocarditis (a biofilm disease), higher doses of antibiotics for longer durations are more successful. However, the growing concern regarding bacteria that are resistant to antibiotic therapy encourages medicine to examine alternative — and possibly better — ways to attack bacterial infections.

It may be ideal to use agents that disrupt the structure of the biofilm infection (*Table 2*). The body's immune system and antibiotics are more successful at destroying individual bacteria cells than destroying biofilm communities of bacteria. Bacteria that are free of their biofilm community are more susceptible to a variety of currently available antimicrobials. This may explain why non-selective biocides (agents that injure the host cell as well as bacteria, such as alcohol, acetic acid, Dakin's solution) are detrimental to wound healing (Wolcott, 2007). Non-selective biocides are more detrimental to host defences and to host healing components than they are to the bacteria. Therefore, clinically relevant agents that specifically target the biofilm need to be developed.

Table 2. Anti-biofilm agents

Agent	Mechanism	Reference
Lactoferrin	Impairs irreversible attachment; ↓ Fe availability	Psaltis et al. (2007) Ward et al. (2002) Weinberg (2007) Singh et al. (2002)
EDTA	Limits attachment; ↓ availability of Fe	Percival et al. (2005)
Xylitol	Impairs matrix development; impairs cell-wall thickening in Gram-positives	Tapiainen et al. (2004) Katsuyama et al. (2005a,b)
Gallium	Disrupts Fe metabolism	Kaneko et al. (2007)
Dispersin B	Impairs matrix by breaking the -1,6 linkage of PNAG	Chaignon et al. (2007) Donelli et al. (2007)
Farnesol	↓ pyocyanin and PQS in *P. aeruginosa* ↓ matrix in *S. aureus*	Katsuyama et al. (2005a,b) Jabra-Rizk et al. (2006)
RNA-III inhibiting peptide (RIP)	Blocks agr expression in *Staphylococcus*	Balaban et al. (2003a,b)
Furanone C30	Quorum-sensing inhibitor in Gram-negatives	Hentzer et al. (2003) Wu et al. (2004)

Many agents have been identified as being useful in interfering with the formation of bacterial biofilms. Some of these agents are listed with their proposed mechanism of action and accompanying references. Not all of these agents are currently used in medicine. FE = iron, EDTA = ethylene diamine tetraacetic acid, PNAG = poly-N-acetylglucosamine, PQS = Pseudomonas quinolone signal

But before these treatments can be pursued fully, we need to understand whether biofilm impairs wound healing at the molecular level and if so, how. The question that begs an answer becomes, 'Is biofilm impairing wound healing or is it just filling a niche?' This question can be answered indirectly by specifically managing biofilm on the surface of chronic wounds. If biofilm management, in combination with standard-of-care management, improves wound-healing outcomes, then this improvement is good indirect evidence that the presence of biofilm is a barrier to wound healing.

We inferred from clinical and laboratory evidence that biofilm may be an important factor that perpetuates the chronicity of non-healing wounds (Wolcott et al., 2008). We began to manage chronic wounds with the assumption that bacterial biofilm was important and needed to be fervently managed in June 2002. We observed anecdotal evidence that this strategy was clinically helpful, and by August 2002 we had begun managing all wounds with the assumption that biofilm is a key component of the wound's pathology.

The role of critical limb ischaemia and comorbidities

This study examines biofilm-based wound care (BBWC) in the context of CLI. Wounds in limbs with poor perfusion are among the most difficult to heal (Marston et al., 2006). Patients with a chronic wound in a diabetic limb with a TCpO$_2$ less than 20mmHg are often managed by major limb amputation. Additional comorbidities such as neuropathy and osteomyelitis often do not come into play. In our clinical experience, CLI in a diabetic patient is sufficient in most physicians' opinions to necessitate a major limb amputation. This reality translates into a near 0% limb salvage rate in such patients.

The healing of wounds, especially in diabetic patients, can be a life-or-death situation. Diabetic patients undergoing a major limb amputation suffer and subsequently die much earlier than their bipedal counterparts. Apelqvist et al. (1993) showed that after a major limb amputation, diabetic patients underwent contralateral limb amputation in 48% of cases within five years. Pohjolainen et al. (1998) demonstrated that the five-year mortality rate for diabetics after a major limb amputation is 80%. Diabetics with wounds, especially wounds with CLI, are facing a very dire situation (Faglia et al., 2006).

Kalani et al. (1999) pursued a study to determine the predictive value of TCpO$_2$ measurements in the outcomes of diabetic foot ulcers. The results suggest that TCpO$_2$ measurements less than 25mmHg carried a very poor prognosis for wound healing. In the study, patients were followed for up to two years, and wounds healed or improved in only two out of 13 patients with CLI. Even though the standard of care was acceptable and included a multidisciplinary team, individualised dressings and offloading, the care did not rise to the standard of current management. The limb salvage rate of only 15% is not surprising.

However, Fife et al.'s (2002) large retrospective study of the correlation of TCpO$_2$ levels to outcomes of hyperbaric oxygen (HBO) management provides more promising results. The standard of care for wound management provided to patients was not described in detail in the paper, but a description of the advanced wound care was provided. Aggressive and frequent debridement, appropriate antibiotics, offloading, advanced dressings, non-invasive vascular assessment, revascularisation as necessary, cell therapies, and HBO were provided in a coordinated multidisciplinary fashion. Fife et al. identified 629 diabetic patients (302 [48%] with critical ischaemia as defined as a TCpO$_2$ below 20mmHg), for whom analysis showed 65% improved or completely re-epithelialised their wounds.

Despite the promising results reported in the literature, patients with CLI who develop wounds are being managed in very different ways, depending solely on which physician they visit first. Some physicians choose immediate amputation in a wounded, critically ischaemic limb; other physicians pursue a trial of therapy. A major and sometimes painful paradigm shift in medicine concerning limb salvage is under way.

In this study, chronic wounds in limbs with CLI were chosen to evaluate the efficacy of BBWC to determine if it can increase the frequency of healing.

Method

The Southwest Regional Wound Care Center in Lubbock, Texas, US performed this retrospective study with institutional review board (IRB) approval through Western IRB (WIRB Protocol No. 20070542; Study No. 1088934). The evaluation period was August 2002 to January 2006. This timeframe closely correlates with the development of anti-biofilm methods, particularly the use of lactoferrin and xylitol as primary anti-biofilm treating agents (Weinberg, 2001, 2007; Ward et al., 2002, 2005; Tapiainen et al., 2004; Psaltis et al., 2007). A total of 4500 unique, wounded patients were screened. Of these, 1400 patients' TCpO$_2$ levels were measured; 266 patients with a TCpO$_2$ less than 20mmHg in their wounded limbs were identified. These were full-thickness wounds of more than 30 days' duration.

Wounds were assessed for the probability of healing in the context of each given patient (eg, end-of-life issues, overwhelming comorbidities). Patients who would not benefit from the risk of aggressive limb salvage were identified and returned to the care of their referring physician; of the 266 patients, 33 had one visit and 17 had two visits before the patients were returned to the referring physician as not acceptable candidates for limb salvage. This resulted in an 'intention-to-treat' group of 216 patients. The intention-to-treat group lost 26 patients before the fourth week (five visits or less) due to the patients or their families deciding not to pursue limb salvage, one death, transportation issues, or other problems. The remaining 190 patients in the treatment group were available for evaluation. Statistical analyses comparing proportions were performed using JMP 6.0 software (SAS Institute).

Each of the 190 patients' records was evaluated for age, sex, presence of diabetes, $TCpO_2$, debridement of bone (osteomyelitis), and the outcome of wound healing. The latter was determined by direct observation or by telephone follow-up. Patients who could not be reached for follow-up were placed into the 'non-healing' group. Wounds that showed or were reported to show complete re-epithelialisation were considered healed; all other wounds were categorised as non-healed. Healing was evaluated in or before March 2007.

Standard care — including clinical assessment of perfusion, nutrition, offloading, and local wound factors — was provided to ensure all clinically relevant barriers to healing were addressed and managed at each visit. The vast majority of visits were at the Wound Care Center on a weekly basis. Non-invasive vascular tests were performed on the first visit, and patients were referred for revascularisation as necessary, although intravascular revascularisation was not available locally until mid-2004.

Patients identified as candidates for limb salvage were managed using a simple biofilm-based wound care (BBWC) algorithm (*Figure 4*). Wounds were debrided using sharp debridement, beginning with the first visit. Ultrasonic debridement (Sonoca, Söring) was used in conjunction with the sharp debridement to manage the surface of the wound as deemed appropriate. The first principle of debridement was to alter the anatomy of the wound by removing surfaces that touch each other (opening all tunnels and removing undermining). The second principle was to remove all devitalised tissue until normal extracellular matrix demonstrating adequate blood supply was reached. All discoloured and soft bone was removed to reveal normal bleeding bone. The debridement of bone was considered sufficient to constitute the diagnosis of osteomyelitis. All slough was removed during debridement.

Clinical methods and agents specifically designed to suppress wound biofilm were instituted in June 2002. The agents chosen to suppress biofilm were identified by talking to biofilm experts and by confirmation in the literature (Singh et al., 2002; Katsuyama et al., 2005a, b). Substances listed by the Food and Drug Administration as Generally Recognised As Safe (GRAS) were considered for standard clinical use. Using agents with a GRAS rating in an off-label manner, yet complementary to standard-of-care management, is believed to be in line with the *Model Guidelines for the Use of Complementary*

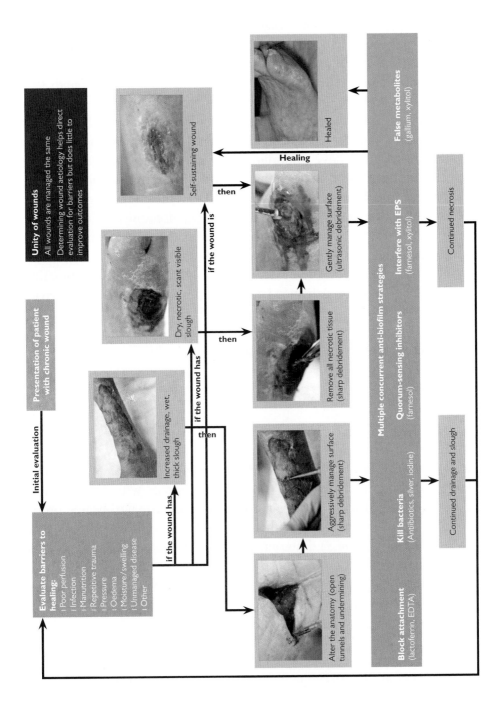

Figure 4. Biofilm-based wound-care algorithm.

and Alternative Therapies in Medical Practice, as approved by the US House of Delegates of the Federation of State Medical Boards (2002).

The primary complementary agents chosen were lactoferrin and xylitol at concentrations of 20mg/cm^3 and 50mg/cm^3 respectively, compounded in a methylcellulose gel. Singh et al. (2002) reported that although low concentrations of lactoferrin did not inhibit growth of planktonic (single cell) *Pseudomonas aeruginosa* cells in culture, lactoferrin did prevent attachment and, therefore, subsequent biofilm formation. Xylitol has also been demonstrated to have important anti-biofilm properties (Katsuyama et al., 2005a, b). Xylitol, in combination with lactoferrin and ionic silver, seem to have important synergies when used to topically manage wounds. Selective biocides, such as silver-impregnated dressings or cadexomer iodine, were used in combination with lactoferrin and xylitol. Non-selective biocides and other agents toxic to host cells were avoided.

Antibiotics were considered an adjunct, being used in combination with the above agents. Advanced technologies such as platelet-derived growth factor-beta, cell therapy (Dermagraft, Advanced Biohealing and Apligraf, Organogenesis), and hyperbaric oxygen (HBO) were used as deemed necessary by the treating clinician.

Results

Of the 190 patients included for evaluation in the study, 146 (77%) showed complete healing and 44 (23%) were categorised as non-healing. The healed group included 47% (68/146) of patients with osteomyelitis and 69% (101/146) with diabetes mellitus, whereas the non-healed group had 75% (33/44) of patients with osteomyelitis and 77% (34/44) with diabetes mellitus (*Table 3*). Photographs of the 190 cases are provided for verification at www.woundcarehospital.com.

The mean age for the healed group was 70.1 years (±13.2) (range 17–95) and 72.4 years (±12.7) (range 43–95) for the non-healed group. The group showing complete healing had 56% males, whereas the non-healing group had 48% males. TCpO$_2$ findings for the successful cohort were 9.3 ± 6.4mmHg (range 0–19) and 6.8 ± 5.7mmHg (range 0–19) for the failed cohort. Thirty-eight patients had wounds that appeared to be moving towards healing but discontinued follow-up (for unknown reasons) before pictures documented complete epithelialisation; 36 of these patients reported healing via telephone. Two patients could not be contacted by

Table 3. Results of biofilm-based wound-care strategies in patients with critically ischaemic wounded limbs

	Healed	Not healed	Total	% healed
All CLI patients	146	44	190	77%
CLI without diabetes or osteomyelitis	30	3	33	91%
CLI and osteomyelitis	68	33	101	67%
CLI and diabetes	101	34	135	75%
CLI with osteomyelitis and diabetes	53	26	79	67%

Under the current standard of care, most of these wounds would have been deemed 'unhealable' and would have resulted in a major limb amputation, but this table demonstrates that the majority of these wounds healed using biofilm-based wound care

telephone and were included in the non-healed category. No treatment complications were reported.

When considering the 216 patients in the intention-to-treat group, the healing rate dropped to 68% (146/216); 20% (44/216) did not heal, and 12% (26/216) did not enter this treatment programme.

Three case histories are provided to illustrate the efficacy of BBWC (*Cases 1–3*, see boxes). All three responded to the use of topical lactoferrin and xylitol in conjunction with other methods, as described in the methodology. One patient required the compassionate use of RNA-III inhibiting peptide (RIP) (Balaban et al., 2003, 2005). RIP is a quorum-sensing inhibitor that interferes with important biofilm pathways in staphylococci. This patient had meticillin-resistant *Staphylococcus aureus* that was recalcitrant to all conventional therapies, requiring innovative biofilm strategies.

Discussion

The 77% healing rate of all the patients with CLI managed in the biofilm-based treatment group is better than the healing rate obtained in patients

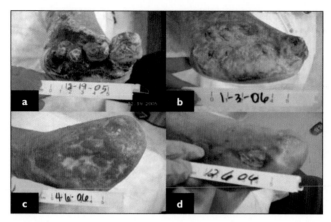

Case 1. The patient is an 84-year-old Hispanic male who presented with progressive necrosis of his right foot. The patient had severe critical limb ischaemia (TCpO₂ of 1mmHg). He presented with multiple medical problems including poor glycaemic control, hypoalbuminaemia, anaemia and concordance issues. The patient was a patriarch of a very large family and decided that he would salvage his foot. He was started on standard wound management along with biofilm-based wound-care strategies in December 2005. The patient received advanced dressings, aggressive and frequent debridement, revascularisation in mid-January 2006, and topical anti-biofilm agents including lactoferrin (20mg/cm³) and xylitol (50mg/ cm³). The patient took over one year to heal, but was able to ambulate on his foot throughout the entire course of healing. Inset d was taken in December 2006, and complete healing was reported in February 2007.

Case 2. This 56-year-old had a history of diabetes for more than two decades. Progressive necrosis of the forefoot developed, beginning with a small traumatic wound of the second toe. By August 2004 major limb amputation was recommended because of the extensive tissue loss of the forefoot. The patient

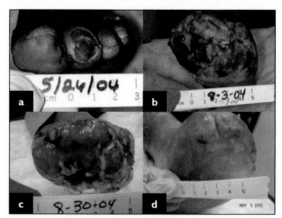

refused amputation. Lactoferrin and RNA-III inhibiting peptide were used as complementary therapies. The change in the wound during the month of August 2004 was dramatic (insets b and c). The change correlates with the addition of anti-biofilm agents to the patient's standard wound-care regimen.

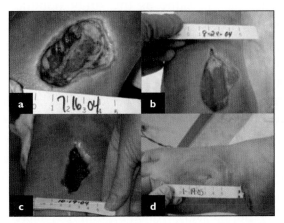

Case 3. This 63-year-old diabetic patient was eight years'post-renal transplant when he developed a wound from a brace applied to his right foot to manage severe Charcot deformity. The wound had eroded into the tarsals of the foot. The patient's $TCpO_2$ was 4mmHg. Lactoferrin ($20mg/cm^3$) was begun in July 2004, which produced immediate improvements in the wound, including decreased drainage, less devitalised tissue, less slough and improved colour and texture in the granulating wound bed. The wound healed in six months.

treated aggressively at other modern wound-care treatment facilities. Even in patients with the combined comorbidities of diabetes and osteomyelitis, healing rates were 67%. Seventy-five per cent of patients with diabetes and CLI healed completely. It is proposed that the improvement in outcomes in these patients over those reported in the literature correlates directly with the use of anti-biofilm agents and methods that were used to manage the wounds. These findings provide indirect evidence that biofilm is indeed an important barrier to wound healing.

The closest match for the patients included in this study with patient populations reported in the literature are those reported in Fife et al.'s (2002) retrospective analysis. Fife reported on 629 diabetic patients, 48% with CLI, whose wounds responded to wound care 65% of the time. For comparison with the current study, we will consider those 65% of subjects to be 'healed'. The patients evaluated in the current study numbered 190 (53% diabetic, 100% with CLI). Only patients with complete healing were included in the 'healed' contingent, which is a more stringent criterion than the 'not failed' category described in Fife et al.'s study.

Although Fife's patient populations are incompletely defined, they are similar enough to investigate statistical comparison, and they received similar wound care to the subjects in the present study, with the exception of BBWC being employed only in the present study.

The null hypothesis used was as follows: the current study

population's healing frequency is the same as the study population reported by Fife ($P_1=P_2$). Using Fisher's exact test ($p<0.05$) and the z-test ($p<0.05$), the null hypothesis must be rejected. Patients healed significantly more frequently using BBWC than using traditional wound care alone (98% confidence).

Biofilm-based wound care also improved the performance of other treatments. For example, we observed an improved clinical response to allograft and xenograft skin, growth factors, and cell therapy. We observed much less degradation of the graft material or the applied growth factors. The 'normal' appearance of graft material at three to five days with a BBWC approach is a much more intact graft instead of the degraded, slimy material that used to be seen (*Figure 5*). Suppressing wound biofilm may increase the efficacy of advanced technologies, such as purified keratinocytes and/or fibroblasts. With less enzymatic degradation and fewer bacterial virulence factors, the applied cells and small proteins seem to work much better.

We deduce that part of the improvement in clinical outcomes when using BBWC is due to a decrease in matrix metalloproteinase activity, decreased elastase activity, and decreased exudate in the wound environment (Wolcott et al., 2008). These characteristics are much more conducive to the effects of growth factors, other applied proteins, and living cells.

Because of this improved clinical efficacy of these proactive healing agents, we have turned to them earlier and in more patients, significantly increasing their use.

Finally, targeting biofilm with anti-biofilm agents can markedly improve the efficacy of antibiotics and HBO therapy. This has led to significant reductions in our use of these interventions, which seems counterintuitive. However, since antibiotics and HBO are operating against disrupted biofilm colony defences, they can achieve their goals in a shorter time. Also, we find that fewer wounds deteriorate to the point that requires these therapies. Over the four years of the study, the use of antibiotics declined by approximately 25% and the use of HBO by 50%. During the same time period the number of actively treated patients increased.

Bacterial biofilm seems to be detrimental to wound healing. In an ischaemic wound where the peri-wound cells are in a desperate struggle for survival, it is not difficult to imagine that the presence of biofilm could easily tip the balance towards cell death and wound deterioration. We have demonstrated that managing wounds as if biofilm were an important barrier to healing improves wound-healing outcomes.

Amputation is a failed strategy. The risk of a trial of therapy to heal

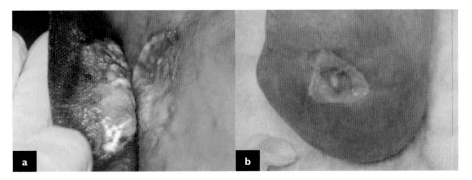

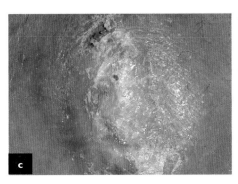

Figure 5. Application of Apligraf without addressing wound biofilm often results in degradation of the graft into a slimy mass after one week (a), possibly due to wound biofilm. By pretreating the wound with anti-biofilm agents and concurrently applying them when the graft is applied (b), Apligraf treatments may lead to more favourable clinical results in as little as one week (c)

the wound and consequently salvage the limb is acceptable in the context of the abysmal results associated with major limb amputation. Under the current standard of care, most of the wounds included in this study would have been deemed 'unhealable' and resulted in a major limb amputation, but with BBWC the majority of these wounds healed.

This study demonstrates that the current standard of care for chronic wounds combined with biofilm-based strategies can achieve a healing frequency of 75% in diabetic patients with critically ischaemic wounded limbs.

The future of biofilm-based wound care

Advances in biofilm treatment are being made. For example, it is difficult to determine biofilm suppression; currently, it can only be assessed clinically. The clinical assessment includes limited slough, scant drainage, and good colour with texture, which are only fair indicators for determining the amount and viability of residual biofilm.

Soon bedside tests will be available to quantify wound bed protease activities, which should be a good surrogate marker for remnant wound biofilm. This is because the protease activities should be proportional to the amount of active biofilm present in the wound.

However, there is much work yet to be done on BBWC. No randomised studies have been performed, and few commercial agents are available that specifically attempt to manage biofilm in chronic wounds.

To our knowledge, this study is the first that goes beyond anecdotal evidence to demonstrate that specifically managing biofilm factors increases favourable wound outcomes. Biofilm-based treatment strategies are in their infancy and need to be developed and tested further, not only to identify key components or combinations of therapy that provide this benefit, but also to identify better agents and combination therapies that further increase the speed or frequency of wound healing.

Additionally, we need better diagnostic tools that are able not only to identify the bacteria in wounds that are culturable, but also the bacteria in wounds that are not culturable (Dowd et al., 2008a, b).

Agents that work to disrupt biofilms need to be studied more fervently:

- Quorum-sensing inhibitors (RIP, furanone C30)
- Agents that degrade the EPS (dispersin B, alginase, phage depolymerases)
- Iron scavengers (EDTA, deferoxamine, transferrins)
- False metabolites (gallium, alcohol sugars)
- A host of ingenious agents produced by plants, animals or microbes themselves.

It is exciting to realise that within a relatively short period of time the clinician could possess a large selection of anti-biofilm agents.

The rational and simultaneous use of these agents along with traditional antimicrobials will likely have additive or synergistic effects on treating biofilm infections.

The authors thank Garth James and the medical biofilm group at the Center for Biofilm Engineering at Montana State University for their excellent work investigating wound biofilm using microscopic and molecular techniques; Scot Dowd for his help in performing the statistical analyses, and Angela Eaton of Texas Tech University for her assistance with editing.

References

Akopian G, Nunnery SP, Piangenti J et al. (2006) Outcomes of conventional wound treatment in a comprehensive wound center. *Am Surg* **72**(4): 314–17

Apelqvist J, Larsson J, Agardh CD (1993) Long-term prognosis for diabetic patients with foot ulcers. J

Intern Med **233**(6): 485–91

Balaban N, Giacometti A, Cirioni O, et al. (2003) Use of the quorum-sensing inhibitor RNAIII-inhibiting peptide to prevent biofilm formation *in vivo* by drug-resistant *Staphylococcus epidermidis. J Infect Dis* **187**(4): 625–30

Balaban N, Stoodley P, Fux CA, et al. (2005) Prevention of staphylococcal biofilm-associated infections by the quorum sensing inhibitor RIP. *Clin Orthop Relat Res* **437**: 48–54

Bjarnsholt T, Kirketerp-Moller K, Jensen PO et al. (2008) Why chronic wounds will not heal; a novel hypothesis. *Wound Repair Regen* **16**(1): 2–10

Chaignon P, Sadovskaya I, Ragunah C, et al. (2007) Susceptibility of staphylococcal biofilms to enzymatic treatments depends on their chemical composition. *Appl Microbiol Biotechnol* **75**(1): 125–32

Costerton JW, Stewart PS, Greenberg EP (1999) Bacterial biofilms: a common cause of persistent infections. *Science* **284**: 1318–22

Donelli G, Francolini I, Romoli D, et al. (2007) Synergistic activity of dispersin B and cefamandole nafate in inhibition of staphylococcal biofilm growth on polyurethanes. *Antimicrob Agents Chemother* **51**(8): 2733–40

Dowd SE, Sun Y, Secor PR et al. (2008a) Survey of bacterial diversity in chronic wounds using Pyrosequencing DGGE, and full ribosome shotgun sequencing. *BMC Microbiol* **8**: 43. www.biomedcentral.com/1471–2180/8/43

Dowd SE, Wolcott RD, Sun Y, McKeehan T, Smith E, Rhoads D (2008b). Polymicrobial nature of chronic diabetic foot ulcer biofilm infections determined using bacterial tag encoded FLX amplicon pyrosequencing (bTEFAP). *PLoS. ONE.* **3**, e3326.

Faglia E, Clerici G, Clerissi J, et al. (2006) Early and five-year amputation and survival rate of diabetic patients with critical limb ischemia: data of a cohort study of 564 patients. *Eur J Vasc Endovasc Surg* **32**(5): 484–90

Federation of State Medical Boards (2002) *Model Guidelines for the Use of Complementary and Alternative Therapies in Medical Practice.* www.fsmb.org/pdf/2002_grpol_Complementary_Alternative_Therapies.pdf

Fife CE, Buyukcakir C, Otto GH, et al. (2002) The predictive value of transcutaneous oxygen tension measurement in diabetic lower extremity ulcers treated with hyperbaric oxygen therapy: a retrospective analysis of 1,144 patients. *Wound Repair Regen* **10**(4): 198–207

Fux CA, Costerton JW, Stewart PS, Stoodley P (2005)Survival strategies of infectious biofilms. *Trends Microbiol* **13**(1): 34–40

Harrison-Balestra C, Cazzaniga AL, Davis SC, Mertz PM (2003) A wound-isolated *Pseudomonas aeruginosa* grows a biofilm *in vitro* within 10 hours and is visualized by light microscopy. *Dermatol Surg* **29**(6): 631–5

Hentzer M, Wu H, Andersen JB, et al. (2003) Attenuation of *Pseudomonas aeruginosa* virulence by quorum sensing inhibitors. *EMBO J* **22**(15): 3803–15

Jabra-Rizk MA, Meiller TF, James CE, Shirtliff ME (2006) Effect of farnesol on *Staphylococcus aureus* biofilm formation and antimicrobial susceptibility. Antimicrob Agents Chemother **50**(4): 1463–9

James G, Swogger E, Wolcott R et al. (2007) Biofilms in chronic wounds. *Wound Repair Regen* **16**(1): 37–44

Kaneko Y, Thoendel M, Olakanmi O, et al. (2007) The transition metal gallium disrupts *Pseudomonas aeruginosa* iron metabolism and has antimicrobial and antibiofilm activity. *J Clin Invest* **117**(4): 877–88

Katsuyama M, Kobayashi Y, Ichikawa H, et al. (2005a) A novel method to control the balance of skin microflora Part 2. A study to assess the effect of a cream containing farnesol and xylitol on atopic dry skin. *J Dermatol Sci* **38**(3): 207–13

Katsuyama M, Ichikawa H, Ogawa S, Ikezawa Z (2005b) A novel method to control the balance of skin microflora. Part 1. Attack on biofilm of *Staphylococcus aureus* without antibiotics. *J Dermatol Sci* **38**(3): 197–205

Leung KP, Crowe TD, Abercrombie JJ et al. (2005) Control of oral biofilm formation by an antimicrobial decapeptide. *J Dent Res* **84**(12): 1172–7

Marston WA, Davies SW, Armstrong B et al. (2006) Natural history of limbs with arterial insufficiency and chronic ulceration treated without revascularization. *J Vasc Surg* **44**(1): 108–14

McIsaac C (2005) Managing wound care outcomes. *Ostomy Wound Manage* **51**(4): 54–6, 58, 59

Mertz PM (2003) Cutaneous biofilms: friend or foe? *Wounds* **15**(5): 1–9

National Institutes of Health (1997) *Minutes of the National Advisory Dental and Craniofacial Research Council* — 153rd Meeting. National Institutes of Health, September 1997. www.nidcr.nih.gov/AboutNIDCR/CouncilAndCommittees/NADCRC/Minutes/Minutes153.htm

Percival SL, Kite P, Eastwood K, et al. (2005) Tetrasodium EDTA as a novel central venous catheter lock solution against biofilm. *Infect Control Hosp Epidemiol* **26**(6): 515–19

Pohjolainen T, Alaranta H (1998) Ten-year survival of Finnish lower limb amputees. *Prosthet Orthot Int* **22**(1): 10–16

Psaltis AJ, Ha KR, Beule AG, et al. (2007) Confocal scanning laser microscopy evidence of biofilms in patients with chronic rhinosinusitis. *Laryngoscope* **117**(7): 1302–6

Reynolds T, Cole E (2006) Techniques for acute wound closure. *Nurs Stand* **20**: 21, 55–64

Sauer K, Camper AK, Ehrlich GD, et al. (2002) *Pseudomonas aeruginosa* displays multiple phenotypes during development as a biofilm. *J Bacteriol* **184**(4): 1140–54

Singh PK, Parsek MR, Greenberg EP, Welsh MJ (2002) A component of innate immunity prevents bacterial biofilm development. *Nature* **417**: 552–5

Tapiainen T, Sormunen R, Kaijalainen T, et al. (2004) Ultrastructure of *Streptococcus pneumoniae* after exposure to xylitol. *J Antimicrob Chemother* **54**(1): 225–8

Ward PP, Uribe-Luna S, Conneely OM (2002) Lactoferrin and host defense. *Biochem Cell Biol* **80**(1): 95–102

Ward PP, Paz E, Conneely OM (2005) Multifunctional roles of lactoferrin: a critical overview. *Cell Mol Life Sci* **62**(22): 2540–8

Weinberg ED (2001) Human lactoferrin: a novel therapeutic with broad spectrum potential. *J Pharm Pharmacol* **53**(10): 1303–10

Weinberg ED (2007) Antibiotic properties and applications of lactoferrin. *Curr Pharm Des* **13**(8): 801–11

Welsh E, Cazzaniga AL, Davis SC, Mertz PM (2003) *Demonstration of Staphylococcus aureus biofilms in acute, partial-thickness wounds in pigs using electron microscopy.* Abstract. Symposium on Advanced Wound Care.

Wolcott RD (2007) Bio-film based wound care. In: Sheffield PJ, Fife CE (eds). *Wound Care Practice* (2nd edn) Best Publishing

Wolcott RD, Rhoads DD, Dowd SE (2008) Biofilms and chronic wound inflammation. *J Wound. Care* **17**: 333-4.

Wu H, Song Z, Hentzer M, et al. (2004) Synthetic furanones inhibit quorum-sensing and enhance bacterial clearance in *Pseudomonas aeruginosa* lung infection in mice. J *Antimicrob Chemother* **53**(6): 1054–61

Bacterial profiling using skin grafting, standard culture and molecular bacteriological methods

A Andersen, K E Hill, P Stephens, D W Thomas, B Jorgensen and K A Krogfelt

It is becoming increasingly apparent that we are experiencing an obesity epidemic. This, coupled with the increase in life expectancy for most Europeans, will result in more patients having chronic diseases, with a consequent increase in complications such as chronic wounds (World Health Organization, 2003).

The prevalence and incidence of leg ulcers, pressure ulcers and diabetic foot ulcers in Denmark is similar to that in the rest of the industrialised world, with about 1% of the Danish population experiencing problem wounds at any one time. Total treatment expenditure for such wounds in Denmark is estimated as being approximately 2–3% of the total health-care system budget (Gottrup, 2004).

The aetiology of chronic leg and foot ulcers is multifactorial when chronic wounds do not progress through the normal phases of wound healing (Nwomeh et al., 1998; Agren et al., 2000). It is now accepted that the bacterial microflora of chronic wounds play a significant role in the impairment of healing. There is also a risk that these wounds will become clinically infected, with the concomitant possibility of other complications such as septicaemia (Bowler, 2003). The detrimental effects of bacterial metabolites, toxins and lysates in the wound environment have been explored (Wall et al., 2002; Ovington et al., 2003; Stephens et al., 2003), with wounds also acting as reservoirs and potentially cross-contaminating sources of antibiotic-resistant microorganisms in hospitals and nursing homes (Day and Armstrong, 1997).

Numerous studies have attempted to establish the microbial component of non-healing wounds, but they have seldom been comparable owing to differences in the microbial sampling and analysis, patient demographics, aetiology and the infection status of the wounds studied (Howell-Jones et al., 2005).

The chronic wound environment is often polymicrobial, the predominant aerobic bacteria isolated from skin wounds being *Staphylococcus aureus*, *Pseudomonas aeruginosa* and coagulase-negative staphylococci (CNS) (Howell-Jones et al., 2005). In addition, anaerobic bacteria constitute a significant proportion of the microbial population in chronic wounds, the most commonly isolated species being Peptostreptococcus and pigmented and non-pigmented Prevotella/Porphyromonas.

The stability and continuity of the microbial community within chronic wounds has not yet been much investigated, although certain species may persist over time, and overall these wounds are perceived to be a dynamically changing environment (Howell-Jones et al., 2005). Recent studies using molecular techniques have demonstrated that chronic wounds harbour a greater bacterial diversity than revealed by culturing alone, and confirmed that denaturing gradient gel electrophoresis (DGGE) as a powerful tool in clinical bacteriology (Hill et al., 2003; Davies et al., 2004). However, it should be noted that Lemmon and Gardner (2008) have suggested caution when interpreting results from these assays as they have found that sensitivities are generally too low for clinical use as real-time polymerase chain reaction (PCR) assays are limited by the quality of the primers and probes chosen. They recommend that the primers and probes must be sensitive enough to match all target organisms yet specific enough to exclude all others.

In addition, depending on the sampling techniques used, numerous studies may have underestimated the population of strict anaerobes within such wounds.

The microbial burden of the wound environment has been characterised as progressing through five stages:

- Contamination
- Colonisation
- Critical colonisation/local infection
- Spreading invasive infection
- Septicaemia.

The emphasis is on the concept of critical colonisation (Schultz et al., 2003), which some have called a transition state between colonisation and invasive wound infection.

In order to study specific bacterial interactions in the wound environment and the events preceding the progression from colonisation to infection, it is important to investigate the *in vivo* spatial distribution and community composition of bacteria in the wound. This progression depends on the relationship between the colonising microorganisms and the host's ability to manage the bioburden of the wound (Robson, 1997). The conditions that denote these transitional states are still not well understood.

Within the microbial wound community, bacteria can act synergistically, so increasing the pathogenic effect. This can be facilitated by, for instance, the generation of chemical micro-niches, which favour the growth of otherwise unviable organisms such as anaerobes, whose fastidious growth requirements may be met by the release of specific essential nutrients by another member of the polymicrobial population, or possibly by direct impairment of the host immune cells (Bowler et al., 2001).

There is increased speculation that, as in other chronic diseases, within the moist wound environment there exists a biofilm of bacteria embedded in a self-secreted extracellular polysaccharide matrix (EPS) (Costerton et al., 1999; Wysocki, 2002). The presence of wound biofilms has been demonstrated in studies of animal-model acute wounds (Harrison-Balestra et al., 2003). Bacteria that grow in a biofilm have been shown to have significantly increased resistance to antibiotic therapy and protection from host defences. This poses a severe problem in the management of wound bioburden.

Recognition that biofilms may play a role in chronic wounds has opened a new area of potential antimicrobial wound management where, in conjunction with standard antibiotic treatments, novel therapies such as the use of quorum-sensing inhibitors to eradicate the potential protective effect of the biofilm may be used (Rasmussen and Givskov, 2006a, b).

Despite the numerous theories on the bacterial ecology in chronic wounds, little is known about the spatial distribution of the microorganisms within the wound environment, with only a few studies in this area (Louie et al., 1976; Sapico et al., 1986).

To our knowledge, no *in vivo* studies on chronic venous leg ulcers have been performed to determine the spatial distribution of microorganisms using both molecular techniques and routine culture.

A regimen widely used at the Copenhagen Wound Healing Centre to treat non-healing venous leg ulcers that have failed to respond to conservative standard compression treatment is ulcer excision, meshed split-skin transplantation and correction of superficial venous insufficiency in the wound (Kjaer et al., 2003).

Skin grafts may be taken from uninjured donor sites on the patient, grown from the patient's skin cells into a dressing (autograft), and applied as a sheet of bioengineered skin from donor cells (allograft) or preserved skin from animals such as pigs (xenograft) (Bromberg and Song, 1965).

Opinions differ as to the efficacy of these procedures. Randomised controlled studies have recently shown that bilayer artificial skin, used in conjunction with compression bandaging, increases the likelihood of healing, but that further research is needed to determine whether other forms of skin grafting improve healing rates of venous ulcers (Jones and Nelson, 2005). Common to all the procedures is the initial wound bed preparation, combined with ulcer excision.

Here, we describe a novel approach whereby multiple samples, using both tissue biopsies and swabs, were obtained from a chronic venous leg ulcer undergoing skin grafting. Using DGGE and routine culture, the semiquantitative spatial distribution of microorganisms within and across the complex environment of a chronic wound was established.

Method

Patient details

Informed patient consent and ethical approval were obtained. A 59-year-old male patient admitted to the Copenhagen Wound Healing Centre, Bispebjerg Hospital, Denmark, voluntarily agreed to participate. Based on histology, clinical revision, Doppler ankle brachial pressure index and clinical microbiological culturing, the patient was diagnosed with a clinically non-infected chronic venous leg ulcer. Conservative standard compression treatment without topical antibiotic administration did not result in healing, so the patient was admitted to the Copenhagen Wound Healing Centre for ulcer excision and meshed split-skin transplantation.

Sample collection

After sedation (medulla spinalis), but before cleansing, administration of antibiotics or other surgical preparation of the ulcer by the surgical team, the surgeon sampled the wound as arranged before the operation.

The wound was positioned longitudinally on the malleolar region. Samples were taken at three sites through the wound (*Figure 1*): from the wound edge (WE, 1) over the central wound bed (WB, 2) to the opposite wound edge (WE, 3). There was a 2cm distance between each sample site.

Two separate samples were taken at each sample site (approximately 0.5cm²), taking the greatest possible care to avoid cross-contamination of blood and tissue from the other sample sites.

Each sample site was first sampled with a sterile charcoal-tipped swab (SSI 40085, Denmark). The swab was immediately transferred to Stuart transport medium (SSI 28733, Denmark). A biopsy was then taken using a 5mm disposable sterile punch biopsy (Produkte für die Medizin AG, Germany) and immediately transferred to Stuart transport medium. Finally, the entire wound surface was swabbed to obtain a total wound microflora sample.

After sampling, the wound bed and lipodermatosclerotic skin surrounding the ulcer were excised to a distance approximately 1cm from the wound edge, leaving the wound bed with healthy bleeding tissue. A split-skin graft taken with a Zimmer dermatome from the anterior part of the contralateral leg was applied and the graft was dressed (Kjaer et al., 2003). Following postoperative compression bandage therapy, the graft took. No ulcer recurrence has since occurred.

Cultural analysis

The biopsy and swab samples were processed in accordance with SSI standard wound culturing procedures as described in a previous study by our

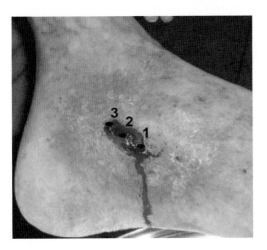

Figure 1. The three sample sites on the chronic venous leg ulcer.

group (Gjødsbøl et al., 2006). All cultured isolates were identified to species level. All initial sample processing (which included plating, preparation for DNA and storage) was done within 80 minutes of sampling.

Tissue DNA extraction

Molecular analysis was undertaken on the tissue samples only. For each extraction, 0.02g of tissue was aseptically dissected longitudinally down the biopsy sample such that each sample contained both wound surface and deep tissue. This was transferred to a sterile microcentrifuge tube. DNA was extracted directly from the tissue, as described by Hill et al. (2003) and stored at –20°C.

DNA extraction from cultured isolates

DNA from pure cultures of the wound isolates was extracted with a QIAmp DNA kit (Qiagen) in accordance with the manufacturer's instructions, and stored at –20°C.

Polymerase chain reaction amplification

The V3 variable region of the 16S rRNA gene was amplified by polymerase chain reaction (PCR) using primers 341f and 518r as previously described (Davies et al., 2004). The previous use of these universal primers is well documented in the literature for amplification of a broad range of bacteria, including their application in a clinical setting (Millar et al., 1996; Schabereiter-Gurtner et al., 2001).

Denaturing gradient gel electrophoresis (DGGE) and sequencing

Denaturing gradient gel electrophoresis was performed using the Bio-Rad DCodeTM Universal Mutation Detection System. Parallel DGGE was performed, essentially as described previously (Davies et al., 2004; Al Soud et al., 2003; Muyzer and Smalla, 1998).

PCR fragments were separated using 9% (w/v) polyacrylamide (acrylamide/bisacrylamide 37.5:1; Bio-Rad) with 10% glycerol, containing a 25–60% linear gradient of denaturants (urea and formamide, Sigma) increasing in the direction of electrophoresis. Polymerase chain reaction samples were applied to gels in aliquots of 35µl per lane, 10µl of DGGE loading buffer (Bio-Rad). The running buffer used was 0.5 x TAE buffer. Electrophoresis was performed at 60°C at 200V for four hours. Gels were stained with SYBR green I (Sigma) diluted in 0.5 x TAE buffer (1:10,000) for 15 minutes and visualised using the Gel Doc 2000 system (Bio-Rad).

The PCR products generated from the cultured isolates were electrophoresised alongside those amplified directly from tissue, allowing for direct comparison between cultured and amplified products from the wound.

The separated DNA fragments were cut from the DGGE gel, extracted and re-amplified using primers 341f and 534r as already described followed by ligation into the pCR4-TOPO vector (Invitrogen, Paisley, UK) and transformation into Top10 competent *Escherichia coli* cells (Invitrogen).

Clones were screened for inserts of the correct size by M13 PCR amplification. DNA for sequencing was prepared from clones using the QIAprep Miniprep kit (Qiagen). Three clones from each excised band were sequenced, and both strands were sequenced at MWG (Germany), using M13f uni (-21) and M13r (-49) primers, giving 100% double coverage of the 193 bp 16S rDNA products for phylogenetic analysis. Sequences obtained were compared with those in the EMBL database (Kulikova et al., 2004) by using FASTA3 (Pearson and Lipman, 1988) at the European Bioinformatics Institute to identify closely related gene sequences. CHIMERA CHECK (Cole et al., 2005) at the RDP was used to detect possible chimeric sequence structures alongside manual inspection of the alignments.

Results

Cultural analysis

The cultured bacterial wound isolates from the three sample sites and the total wound surface swab were identified to species level (*Table 1*). All three sites (*Figure 1*) contained *Staphylococcus aureus*. Sites 1 and 2 also contained *Escherichia coli* and site 3 contained the coagulase-negative *Staphylococcus lugdunensis*. All three species were also cultured from the total wound surface swab (*Table 1*).

DGGE

The DGGE profiles of PCR-amplified pure cultures isolated from the

Table 1. Bacterial identification from different biopsy sites for the same wound identified by culture analysis and DGGE

Biopsy site	Cultured isolates	DGGE
WE 1	*Staphylococcus aureus*	*Staphylococcus aureus*
	Escherichia coli	*Escherichia coli*
WE 2	*Staphylococcus aureus*	*Staphylococcus aureus*
	Escherichia coli	*Escherichia coli*
WE 3	*Staphylococcus aureus*	*Staphylococcus aureus*
	Staphylococcus lugdunensis	
Total wound surface	*Staphylococcus aureus* *Escherichia coli* *Staphylococcus lugdunensis*	

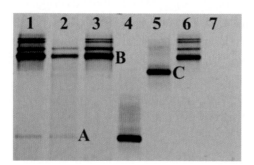

Lanes:
1 Biopsy site 1 (WE 1)
2 Biopsy site 2 (WB 2)
3 Biopsy site 3 (WE 3)
4 *Escherichia coli*
5 *Staphyloccocus lugdunensis*
6 *Staphylococcus aureus*
7 Negative control using Milli-Q water as PCR template.
Bands marked with capital letters were excised, cloned and sequenced

Figure 2. DGGE analysis of 16S rRNA fragments from tissue biopsies from the three sample sites (lanes 1–3) compared with those amplified from cultured isolates from the same wound (lanes 4–6).

wound and the three tissue biopsy sites were compared (*Figure 2*). All biopsy sites had bands corresponding to those obtained from the pure culture isolates. In the *Staphylococcus aureus* pure cultures (lane 6), three distinct extra bands were present above the dominant band. This was also the case in initial gels of the cultured isolates.

To verify the authenticity of this banding pattern for this *Staphylococcus aureus* strain, cells were regrown from frozen cultures and verified on plates as pure cultures of *Staphylococcus aureus*. DNA extraction was repeated and 16S rRNA re-amplified. The banding patterns obtained corresponded exactly to those obtained previously and were similar to the profile from the tissue biopsies.

As all biopsy site sample PCRs were performed using standard concentrations of target DNA, the profiles can be regarded as semiquantitative, as reported by Brüggemann et al. (2000) assuming that the ratio of human to prokaryotic DNA does not change significantly between samples.

The intensities of the bands indicate that *Staphylococcus aureus* was the predominant microorganism in this particular wound environment. The profiles indicate that the cultural analysis may have overestimated the presence of *Staphylococcus lugdunensis* as it did not appear in the DGGE profiles amplified from the three biopsy samples. *Escherichia coli* was identified at two biopsy sites (sites 1 and 2), and band intensities indicate that significantly fewer *Escherichia coli* cells were present in the wound environment compared with *Staphylococcus aureus*.

Sequencing

Although identical migration banding patterns were obtained for the pure culture isolates compared with those from the biopsies (*Figure 2*), we further verified the identity of the species by sequencing bands from the tissue samples or, in the case of *Staphylococcus lugdunensis,* the DGGE band from the pure culture isolate (*Figure 2*).

Discussion and limitations

In this study we have presented novel means for obtaining multiple *in vivo* samples from wounds for the further elucidation of the complex microbiological environment present within chronic venous leg ulcers and other type of wounds suitable for skin grafting. Furthermore, we have demonstrated the combination of standard culture methods and the use of PCR and subsequent DGGE analysis to show the spatial distribution of microorganisms in a chronic venous leg ulcer. In a recent study we demonstrated that the microbial communities in chronic venous leg ulcers can consist of two to 15 different bacterial species

(Gjødsbøl et al., 2006). This emphasises the need to apply molecular techniques to resolve the spatial community distribution.

A superficial swab sample provides a general picture of the wound community, but may increase the number of false positive results (Bowler, 2003; Schultz et al., 2003), whereas tissue biopsy samples are highly localised and may not reflect the microflora in other parts of the wound.

Our results show both scenarios. The swab samples may have overestimated the presence of *Staphylococcus lugdunensis* at site 3 as it did not turn up in the DGGE results. The swab could have been contaminated, but as the utmost care was taken during the sampling, in particular to avoid cross-contamination, it is more likely that the culture conditions favoured a few viable *Staphylococcus lugdunensis*, present at site 3, revealing them in the culture analysis. The bacteria may have been present in numbers below the detection limit of the DGGE and were therefore not detected.

The biopsies showed spatial differences with regard to the presence of *Escherichia coli* at sites 1 and 2 and site 3 (*Figure 2* and *Table 1*). These biopsy results were consistent with the local swab results, confirming that swab and biopsy samples were comparable, as demonstrated by Gjødsbøl et al. (2006) and Davies et al. (2007). DGGE showed a quantitative difference between the three biopsy sites and indicated that the centre of the wound harboured fewer cells of *Staphylococcus aureus* than the two other sampling sites. The presence of three distinct extra bands (above the dominant band) for *Staphylococcus aureus* pure culture (*Figure 2*, lane 6) is an indication of the presence of multiple rrN operons, a phenomenon also reported in other studies (Schabereiter-Gurtner et al., 2001; Al Soud et al., 2003; Davies et al., 2004).

DGGE provides a valuable method of detecting the unculturable fraction of the wound microflora (Davies et al., 2004), although in this particular wound no unculturable organisms were identified. However, DGGE has other potential benefits, as it can identify hard-to-culture wound microflora fractions such as anaerobes, which are often underestimated (Bowler and Davies, 1999). In this study, no anaerobic species were cultured from the wound, as confirmed by DGGE. Hence, although DGGE did not yield any additional information to that obtained from cultural analysis, it is a useful adjunct, validating its use as an appropriate clinically relevant back-up/confirmation of standard laboratory procedures.

Combined use of the sample techniques presented here, utilising culture analysis with DGGE, provides a possibility for assigning bacterial species believed to be detrimental to the wound healing process to different parts, and possibly tissue types, of the wound in further studies. Moreover, this study shows that it is possible to obtain multiple chronic wound samples from a single wound in patients admitted for skin grafting. Since the wound is to be surgically removed, acquiring biopsy samples before surgery does not interfere with any wound healing. Importantly, as the patient is sedated, the procedure does not cause discomfort. In addition, it does not interfere with the surgical procedure if well coordinated with the anaesthetist, surgeon and surgical team.

For this sampling procedure to be possible, a series of factors needs to be in place. The microbiology laboratory responsible for the further analysis of the samples must be fairly close by. This will facilitate good communication with the surgical team and the surgeon in charge when a suitable wound becomes available, which often happens at short notice. Close proximity will also enable samples to be readily collected and quickly processed. Photographing the wound before and after sampling is very helpful in defining appropriate sample sites. This should be done alongside acetate tracings of the wound, a standard procedure in the monitoring and recording of such wounds.

A disadvantage of the sampling technique used in this study, where the whole ulcer bed is subsequently removed, is that it precludes the possibility of a longitudinal study of the wound. This would be possible only if the ulcer recurred and required additional surgery. The bacterial flora of leg ulcers of different aetiologies have been shown to influence the success rate of skin grafting (Gilliland et al., 1988; Unal et al., 2005), and ulcer recurrence is observed. Despite this, treatment with ulcer excision, meshed split-skin transplantation and correction of superficial venous insufficiency in the wound area have shown beneficial results irrespective of the underlying pattern of venous insufficiency (Kjaer et al., 2003). Skin grafting, therefore, poses an excellent opportunity for obtaining multiple insights into the complex bacterial microenvironments that comprise a chronic wound. In most cases, this provides successful treatment to an otherwise non-healing wound, as was the case for this patient.

Conclusion and recommendations

This study has demonstrated that spatial and quantitative differences in the microbiological environment exist within chronic venous leg ulcers and has presented a novel means of obtaining multiple biopsies from a single wound which could be applied to future studies into the *in vivo* spatial distribution of wound microorganisms. It has also verified that DGGE is a powerful and rapid tool for elucidating the clinical microbiology of a chronic disease state.

References

Agren MS, Eaglstein WH, Ferguson MW et al. (2000) Causes and effects of the chronic inflammation in venous leg ulcers. *Acta Derm Venereol Suppl (Stockh)* **210**: 3–17

Al Soud WA, Bennedsen M, On SL et al. (2003) Assess-ment of PCR-DGGE for the identification of diverse Helicobacter species, and application to faecal samples from zoo animals to determine Helicobacter prevalence. *J Med Microbiol* **52**(Pt 9): 765–71

Bowler PG (2003) The 10(5) bacterial growth guideline: reassessing its clinical relevance in wound healing. *Ostomy Wound Manage* 49(1): 44–53

Bowler PG, Davies BJ (1999) The microbiology of infected and noninfected leg ulcers. *Int J Dermatol* **38**(8): 573–8

Bowler PG, Duerden BI, Armstrong DG (2001) Wound microbiology and associated approaches to wound management. *Clin Microbiol Rev* **14**(2): 244–69

Bromberg BE, Song IC (1965) Pigskin heterografts. *Minn Med* **48**(12): 1605–9

Bruggemann J, Stephen JR, Chang YJ et al. (2000) Competitive PCR-DGGE analysis of bacterial mixtures: an internal standard and an appraisal of template enumeration accuracy. *J Microbiol Methods* **40**(2): 111–23

Cole JR, Chai B, Farris RJ et al. (2005) The Ribosomal Database Project (RDP-II): sequences and tools for high-throughput rRNA analysis. *Nucleic Acids Res* **33**(Database issue): D294–D296

Costerton JW, Stewart PS, Greenberg EP (1999) Bacterial biofilms: a common cause of persistent infections. *Science* **284**: 1318–22

Davies CE, Hill KE, Newcombe RG et al. (2007) A prospective study of the microbiology of chronic venous leg ulcers to reevaluate the clinical predictive value of tissue biopsies and swabs. *Wound Repair Regen* **15**(1): 17–22

Davies CE, Hill KE, Wilson MJ et al. (2004) Use of 16S ribosomal DNA PCR and denaturing gradient gel electrophoresis for analysis of the microfloras of healing and nonhealing chronic venous leg ulcers. *J Clin Microbiol* **42**(8): 3549–57

Day MR, Armstrong DG (1997) Factors associated with methicillin resistance in diabetic foot infections. *J Foot Ankle Surg* **36**(4): 322–5

Gilliland EL, Nathwani N, Dore CJ, Lewis JD (1988) Bacterial colonisation of leg ulcers and its effect on the success rate of skin grafting. *Ann R Coll Surg Engl* **70**(2): 105–8

Gjødsbøl K, Christensen J, Karlsmark T et al. (2006) Multiple bacterial species reside in chronic wounds: a longitudinal study. *International Wound Journal* **3**(3): 225–31

Gottrup F (2004) A specialized wound-healing center concept: importance of a multidisciplinary department structure and surgical treatment facilities in the treatment of chronic wounds. *Am J Surg* **187**(5(A)) 38S–43S

Harrison-Balestra C, Cazzaniga AL, Davis SC, Mertz PM (2003) A wound-isolated *Pseudomonas aeruginosa* grows a biofilm in vitro within 10 hours and is visualized by light microscopy.

Dermatol Surg **29**(6): 631–5

Hill KE, Davies CE, Wilson MJ et al. (2003) Molecular analysis of the microflora in chronic venous leg ulceration. *J Med Microbiol* **52**(Pt 4): 365–9

Howell-Jones RS, Wilson MJ, Hill KE et al. (2005) A review of the microbiology, antibiotic usage and resistance in chronic skin wounds. *J Antimicrob Chemother* **55**(2): 143–9

Kjaer ML, Jorgensen B, Karlsmark T et al. (2003) Does the pattern of venous insufficiency influence healing of venous leg ulcers after skin transplantation? *Eur J Vasc Endovasc Surg* **25**(6): 562–7

Kulikova T, Aldebert P, Althorpe N et al. (2004) The EMBL Nucleotide Sequence Database. *Nucleic Acids Res* **32**(Database issue): D27–D30

Jones JE, Nelson EA (2005) Skin grafting for venous leg ulcers. *Cochrane Database Syst Rev* **1**: CD001737

Lemmon GH, Gardner SN (2008) Predicting the sensitivity and specificity of published real-time PCR Assays. *Annals of Clinical Microbiology and Antimicrobials* **7**:18 available at www.ann-clinmicrob.com/content/7/1/18

Louie TJ, Bartlett JG, Tally FP, Gorbach SL (1976) Aerobic and anaerobic bacteria in diabetic foot ulcers. *Ann Intern Med* **85**(4): 461–3

Millar MR, Linton CJ, Cade A et al. (1996) Application of 16S rRNA gene PCR to study bowel flora of preterm infants with and without necrotizing enterocolitis. *J Clin Microbiol* **34**(10): 2506–10

Muyzer G, Smalla K (1998) Application of denaturing gradient gel electrophoresis (DGGE) and temperature gradient gel electrophoresis (TGGE) in microbial ecology. *Antonie Van Leeuwenhoek* **73**(1): 127–41

Nwomeh BC, Yager DR, Cohen IK (1998) Physiology of the chronic wound. *Clin Plast Surg* **25**(3): 341–56

Ovington L et al. (2003) Bacterial toxins and wound healing. *Ostomy Wound Manage* **49**(7A) Suppl: 8–12

Pearson WR, Lipman DJ (1988) Improved tools for biological sequence comparison. *Proc Natl Acad Sci* USA **85**(8): 2444–8

Rasmussen TB, Givskov M (2006a) Quorum sensing inhibitors: a bargain of effects. *Microbiology* **152**(Pt 4): 895–904

Rasmussen TB, Givskov M (2006b) Quorum-sensing inhibitors as anti-pathogenic drugs. *Int J Med Microbiol* **296**(2–3): 149–61

Robson MC (1997) Wound infection. A failure of wound healing caused by an imbalance of bacteria. *Surg Clin North Am* **77**(3): 637–50

Sapico FL, Ginunas VJ, Thornhill-Joynes M et al. (1986) Quantitative microbiology of pressure sores in different stages of healing. *Diagn Microbiol Infect Dis* **5**(1): 31–8

Schabereiter-Gurtner C, Maca S, Rolleke S et al. (2001) 16S rDNA-based identification of bacteria from conjunctival swabs by PCR and DGGE fingerprinting. *Invest Ophthalmol Vis Sci* **42**(6): 1164–71

Schultz GS, Sibbald RG, Falanga V et al. (2003) Wound bed preparation: a systematic approach to wound management. *Wound Repair Regen* **11**(Suppl 1): S1–S28

Stephens P, Wall IB, Wilson MJ et al. (2003) Anaerobic cocci populating the deep tissues of chronic wounds impairs cellular wound healing responses in vitro. *Br J Dermatol* **148**(3): 456–66

Unal S, Ersoz G, Demirkan F et al. (2005) Analysis of skin-graft loss due to infection: infection-related graft. loss *Ann Plast Surg* **55**(1): 102–6

Wall IB, Davies CE, Hill KE et al. (2002) Potential role of anaerobic cocci in impaired human wound healing. *Wound Repair Regen* **10**(6): 346–53

World Health Organization (2003) *Diet, Nutrition and the Prevention of Chronic Diseases.* WHO, Geneva

Wysocki AB (2002) Evaluating and managing open skin wounds: colonization versus infection. *AACN Clin Issues* **13**(3): 382–97

The influence of essential oils on the process of wound healing: a review of the current evidence

A C Woollard, K C Tatham and S Barker

The management of wounds over the millennia of medical history reads like a catalogue of human ingenuity, a combination of trial and error, word of mouth and quizzical speculation. Since Flemming stumbled across the mould that changed the face of mankind's battle with infection, antibiotics have been a mainstay of the treatment of infected wounds. However, they only help to combat one of the factors that prevent wounds from healing instead of truly accelerating the speed of tissue recovery. As we approach an era when pathogens are increasingly immune to our arsenal of antibiotics and their ability to mutate (Erb et al., 2007) is outstripping our inventiveness in creating new ones, many 'forgotten' remedies are once again gaining appeal.

Increasingly, so-called 'natural' approaches to wound management are finding favour within medical, paramedical and lay communities alike. A multimillion dollar industry is also backing these treatments and propelling them into the mainstream. In this review we try to ascertain whether there is any evidence to support the use of some of the more common remedies based on essential oils. We aimed to answer the following questions: Do they have any identifiable benefits in wound healing? Can they be shown to have antimicrobial activity? Are they harmful?

Medline, EMBASE, Cinahl, Allied and Complementary Medicine, and The British Nursing Index were searched using the terms 'essential oils' and 'wound healing or wound care'. Limiting the search to the last 20 years yielded 103 articles.

Wound healing

A wound can be defined as any break in the continuity of the skin that can arise from a myriad of causes ranging from surgery and trauma, to breakdown following pressure. Once a wound is present, the body will naturally begin a process of repair, which occurs in three stages:

ı   The lag phase: an initial phase, which lasts for two to three days, characterised by an inflammatory response. There is an increase in local capillary permeability, resulting in an exudate of serous fluid and inflammatory cells

ı   The incremental phase: angiogenesis results in new capillary buds designed to deliver oxygen and other nutrients to the metabolically active injury site. Fibroblasts and myofibroblasts migrate into the wound to produce collagen and myofibrils respectively. The synthesis of new collagen far exceeds the breakdown of old collagen and, as it accumulates over approximately three weeks, it exponentially increases tensile strength. Myofibrils are responsible for wound contraction, reducing the size of the defect. Capillary buds, combined with fibroblasts, macrophages and leucocytes, make up the red, friable 'granulation tissue' associated with wound healing by secondary intention

ı   The maturation phase: the number of inflammatory cells and fibroblasts declines during this period and the ratio of collagen synthesis:breakdown levels off. Collagen fibres align themselves according to mechanical forces and their tensile strength continues to increase gradually for up to six months. However, the skin will only ever reach approximately 80% of its original strength.

The appearance of the scar changes over time. It becomes steadily redder, more raised and thickened after two weeks in the first three months. It can remain unchanged for as long as a further three months before slowly fading and becoming less prominent. However, the final appearance depends on a myriad of factors including the extent and nature of the injury, age, sex, race, the direction of scar, comorbidities, smoking and infection. Similarly, wound healing is influenced by both general and local factors, which often overlap.

Age, comorbidities, nutritional status and blood supply can all conspire in creating an environment that is unable to cope with the metabolic demands of wound healing. In addition, these same factors, and often treatments such as steroids or radiotherapy for example, can increase the likelihood of wound infection (Mehrabi et al., 2006). A wound that has a good blood supply can usually combat bacterial colonisation through the body's normal defences. However, in a heavily contaminated wound, or one where nutritional supply is poor, infection becomes a major factor in delayed healing.

Surgical technique can have a significant impact on wound healing whether it is the primary cause of the injury or an adjunct to its management (Mehrabi et al., 2006). Asepsis, gentle tissue handling, planning incisions to relieve wound tension, the choice of suture material, haemostasis and judicious use of diathermy all contribute to the speed of healing and final cosmetic result.

Very few of the articles identified in the review produced statistically significant data supporting the use of essential oils in the clinical setting. However, some common trends in the application of these oils to promote wound healing did become apparent across the studies.

Lavender oil

Lavendula (lavender) oil has been used to treat bites, for its antibacterial and antifungal properties, and as an antidepressant and smooth muscle relaxant. Cavanagh and Wilkinson claimed in a review in 2002 that a multitude of data support the use of the various Lavendula species, although this mostly remains 'controversial and inconclusive'. Furthermore, Kane et al. (2004) claimed that lavender oil aromatherapy during dressing changes of vascular wounds significantly reduced subsequent pain intensity when compared with control therapies.

Prashar et al. (2004) studied the cytotoxicity of the oil's components. They demonstrated that two of the oil's components, linalool and linalyl acetate, in equivalent concentrations to that in the lavender oil had cytotoxic effects on human cells *in vitro*. The linalool was equivalent to the effects of whole oil, while the linalyl acetate was more cytotoxic, suggesting that its activity might be suppressed by another component of the oil.

Evandri et al. (2005) analysed the chemical composition of lavender oil using gas chromatography and assessed its antimutagenic activity using bacterial reverse mutation assay. At its maximum concentration, it exhibited strong activity in reducing the number of histidine-independent revertant (mutant) colonies by 66.4% — a property the authors claim makes it a promising candidate for new applications in human health care.

In 2002 Hartman and Coetzee reported the effect of lavender and chamomile on wound healing in a five patients with chronic wounds of three to four months' duration. The wounds were graded using the US National Pressure Ulcer Advisory Panel (NPUAP) guidelines based on depth and visual characteristics, and were treated with a 6% solution of two drops of lavender oil and one drop of German chamomile applied directly to the wound and added to the dressing (gauze/Telfa [Kendall Company]). The wounds treated with the oils healed more quickly than the controls.

Chamomile oil

The evidence for use of chamomile oil is not only exhibited by the previous reference but has also been investigated by Maiche et al. (1991), who studied the effect of chamomile cream and almond ointment on acute radiation skin reactions but they could not demonstrate any benefits. In a German study Glowania et al. (1987) conducted a double-blind trial of 14 patients in which chamomile oil, when added to standard dressings, significantly improved the weeping and drying associated with dermabrasion wounds. In a review of the bioactivity of chamomile, McKay and Blumberg (2006) found it showed moderate antimicrobial and significant antiplatelet activity *in vitro*, as well as anti-mutagenic effects in animals.

Tea tree oil

Melaleuca (tea tree) oil is a popular complementary therapy originating from Australia, which many regard as an effective antiseptic, antibacterial, antifungal and anti-inflammatory agent.

Halcon and Milkus (2004) reviewed the use of tea tree oil as an antimicrobial agent to treat *Staphylococcus aureus*. They claim a benefit of tea tree oil in osteomyelitis and chronic wound healing, but only in small clinical trials and case studies.

Hammer et al. (1996) investigated the efficacy of tea tree oil against transient and commensal skin flora *in vitro*. Comparing concentrations for bactericidal action, it was found to be active against *Staphylococcus aureus* and most Gram-negative bacteria (0.25%) but less effective against coagulase-negative staphylococci and micrococci (8%).

Sherry et al. (2001) claimed that Polytoxinol (Polytoxinol Antimicrobials), an antimicrobial preparation from phytochemical extract of tea tree oil and eucalyptus, was responsible for activity against methicillin-resistant *Staphylococcus aureus* (MRSA) in a case study reported in Australia. This concerns a single case of an adult male with intractable MRSA infection of the tibia that resolved with three months of percutaneously applied treatment into the bone. Carson and Riley (2003) have named tea tree oil as a treatment for skin infections.

Another group in Australia, Faoagali et al. (1997), described the activity of tea tree oil in Burnaid cream (Rye Pharmaceuticals) against *Enterococcus faecalis*, *Staphylococcus aureus*, *Escherichia coli* and *Pseudomonas aeruginosa*, although it was not found to be active against *Enterococcus faecalis* or *Pseudomonas aeruginosa*. They inoculated horse-agar plates with the organisms and then placed samples of Burnaid or base product in wells cut into the agar. Unfortunately, they were unable to show any significant difference between the base constituent and Burnaid antibacterial actions. They went on to state that, in view of evidence they had found describing cytotoxicity of tea tree oil against human fibroblasts and epithelial cells, they could not recommend its use in burns.

Farnan et al. (2005) studied susceptibility to tea tree oil of organisms causing otitis externa, and found 71% of pathogenic organisms cultured were sensitive to it.

Thyme oil

Thymus oil, derived from the herb thyme, has been widely reported to contribute to the healing of burns.

Dursun et al. (2003) investigated this property and the impact of thyme oil on nitric oxide, an important inflammatory mediator in burns injury. Their aim was to elicit any potential protective action of thyme oil on burns-induced nitric oxide production. They burned rats under anaesthesia, and with the inclusion of controls, found that nitric oxide was overproduced by thermal injury. They went on to demonstrate that thyme oil not only decreased the amount nitric oxide produced in response to burns injury but also facilitated wound healing.

Several other studies, such as that by Bozin et al. (2006), have showed significant antibacterial and antifungal actions of thyme oil *in vitro*. This is supported by a similar study by Shin and Kim (2005), which exhibited significant inhibitory action against both antibiotic-susceptible and resistant strains of *Streplococci, Pneumoniae, Staphylococcus aureus* and *Salmonella typhimurium*. Furthermore, Giordani et al. (2004) found that thyme oil significantly potentiates the antifungal action of amphotericin B. The presence in the culture medium of essential oil from *Thymus vulgaris* thymol chemotype (0.01, 0.1, 0.2, 0.3mcg/ml) and amphotericin B decreased the minimum inhibitory concentration (MIC) 80% of amphotericin B. Komarcevic (2000) commented on the evidence that extracts from thyme oil, when topically applied, increased collagen deposition, angiogenesis and keratinocyte migration in wound healing.

Ocimum oil (basil)

Orafidiya et al. (2003) compared *Ocimum gratissimum Linn* (basil) with two commercial topical agents (Cicatrin, GlaxoWellcome and Cetavlex, AstraZeneca) in the healing of full-thickness excisional and incisional wounds created under anaesthesia in rats. They found marked enhancement in wounds treated with the essential oil in comparison with control and reference products.

In 2001 Orafidiya et al. demonstrated the marked antiseptic effects of 2% Ocimum oil against strains and isolates from boils, wounds and acne.

Singh and Majumdar (1999) found that Ocimum oil significantly inhibited enhancement of vascular permeability and leucocyte migration following inflammatory stimulus in animal studies. In a different study Singh (1999) also concluded that *Ocimum basilicum* may be a useful anti-inflammatory agent which blocks both cyclooxygenase and lipoxygenase pathways of the arachidonic acid metabolism.

Other oils

Less well-known essential oils exhibiting similar effects to the above include the bark oil of Santiria (a member of the frankincense family). Martins et al. (2003) described how this oil, used in wound healing in Sao Tome and Principe, is active in culture against several bacterial and fungal strains, especially *Proteus vulgaris* and *Cryptococcus neoformans*.

Lavagna et al. (2001) studied the healing of Caesarean section wounds following application of a mixture of oily extracts of *Hypericum perforatum* (St John's Wort) and *Calendula arvensis* (field marigold).

Kamath et al. (2003) administered oil extracted from *Cinnamomum zeylanicum* (cinnamon) bark to Wistar rats. Given orally at one-quarter or one-eighth LD_{50} it significantly enhanced the tensile strength of incisional wounds, the rate of wound contraction and the period of epithelialisation.

Phan et al. (1998) demonstrated the role of eupolin ointment, an extract from *Chromolaena odorata* (Siam weed), following its use by Vietnamese practitioners on wounds and burns. They showed a significant increase in endothelial and fibroblast cell growth in *in vitro* models, supporting previous studies indicating a role for eupolin in wound remodelling as well as its anticoagulant and antibacterial properties.

Conclusion

A moderately comprehensive search of the literature unearthed surprisingly few papers exploring the role of essential oils in wound healing, and in those found there was a disappointing lack of scientific method to support their hypotheses. However, there does seem to be a general trend suggesting that essential oils possess healing properties, and there are the beginnings of an understanding as to which elements of their make-up might hold the keys to those benefits. It would appear from the general weight of opinion that essential oils have the potential to play a significant role in wound healing. However, at present this is not freely supported by robust clinical trials. In this age of evidence-based medicine, particularly with the current popularity of complementary remedies, it is vital that further, carefully planned, trials take place to confirm their role in modern wound management.

References

Bozin B, Mimica-Dukic N, Simin N, Anackov G (2006) Characterization of the volatile composition of essential oils of some lamiaceae spices and the antimicrobial and antioxidant activities of the entire oils. *J Agric Food Chem* **54**(5): 1822–8

Carson CF, Riley TV (2003) Non-antibiotic therapies for infectious diseases. *Commun Dis Intell* **27**(Suppl): S143–6

Cavanagh HM, Wilkinson JM (2002) Biological activities of lavender essential oil. *Phytother Res*

16(4): 301–8

Dursun N, Liman N, Ozyazgan I et al. (2003) Role of thymus oil in burn wound healing. *J Burn Care Rehabil* **24**(6): 395–9

Erb A, Sturmer T, Marre R, Brenner H (2007) Prevalence of antibiotic resistance in *Escherichia coli*: overview of geographical, temporal, and methodological variations. *Eur J Clin Microbiol Infect Dis* **26**(2): 83–90

Evandri MG, Battinelli L, Daniele C et al. (2005) The anti-mutagenic activity of *Lavandula angustifolia* (lavender) essential oil in the bacterial reverse mutation assay. *Food Chem Toxicol* **43**(9): 1381–7

Faoagali J, George N, Leditschke JF (1997) Does tea tree oil have a place in the topical treatment of burns. *Burns* **23**(4): 349–51

Farnan TB, McCallum J, Awa A et al. (2005) Tea tree oil: *in vitro* efficacy in otitis externa. *J Laryngol Otol* **119**(3): 198–201

Giordani R, Regli P, Kalousti, J et al. (2004) Antifungal effect of various essential oils against *Candida albicans*. Potentiation of antifungal action of amphotericin B by essential oil from *Thymus vulgaris*. *Phytother Res* **18**(12): 990–5

Glowania HJ, Raulin C, Swoboda M (1987) Effect of chamomile on wound healing: a clinical double-blind study. *Z Hautkr* **62**(17): 1262, 1267–71

Halcon L, Milkus K (2004) Staphylococcus aureus and wounds: a review of tea tree oil as a promising antimicrobial. *Am J Infect Control* **32**(7): 402–8

Hammer KA, Carson CF, Riley TV (1996) Susceptibility of transient and commensal skin flora to the essential oil of *Melaleuca alternifolia* (tea tree oil). *Am J Infect Control* **24**(3): 186–9

Hartman D, Coetzee JC (2002) Two US practitioners' experience of using essential oils for wound care. *J Wound Care* **11**(8): 317–20

Kamath JV, Rana AC, Chowdhury AR (2003) Pro-healing effect of *Cinnamomum zeylanicum* bark. *Phytother Res* **17**(8): 970–2

Kane FM, Brodie EE, Coull A et al. (2004) The analgesic effect of odour and music upon dressing change. *Br J Nurs* **13**(19): S4–12

Komarcevic A (2000) [The modern approach to wound treatment.] *Med Pregl* **53**(7–8): 363–8

Lavagna SM, Secci D, Chimenti P et al. (2001) Efficacy of Hypericum and Calendula oils in the epithelial reconstruction of surgical wounds in childbirth with caesarean section. *Farmaco* **56**(5–7): 451–3

Maiche AG, Grohn P, Maki-Hokkonen H (1991) Effect of chamomile cream and almond ointment on acute radiation skin reaction. *Acta Oncol* **30**(3): 395–6

Martins AP, Salgueiro LR, Goncalves MJ et al. (2003) Essential oil composition and antimicrobial activity of *Santiria trimera* bark. *Planta Med* **69**(1): 77–9

McKay DL, Blumberg JB (2006) A review of the bioactivity and potential health benefits of chamomile tea (*Matricaria recutita L.*). *Phytother Res* **20**(7): 519–30

Mehrabi A, Fonouni H, Wente M et al. (2006) Wound complications following kidney and liver transplantation. *Clin Transplant* **20**(Suppl 17): 97–110

Orafidiya LO, Agbani EO, Abereoje OA et al. (2003) An investigation into the wound-healing properties of essential oil of *Ocimum gratissimum linn*. *J Wound Care* **12**(9): 331–4

Orafidiya LO, Oyedele AO, Shittu AO, Elujoba AA et al. (2001) The formulation of an effective topical anti-bacterial product containing *Ocimum gratissimum* leaf essential oil. *Int J Pharm* **224**(1–2): 177–83

Phan TT, Hughes MA, Cherry GW (1998) Enhanced proliferation of fibroblasts and endothelial cells treated with an extract of the leaves of *Chromolaena odorata*, a herbal remedy for treating wounds. *Plast Reconstr Surg* **101**(3): 756–65 Prashar A, Locke IC, Evans CS (2004) Cytotoxicity of lavender oil and its major components to human skin cells. *Cell Prolif* **37**(3): 221–9

Sherry E, Boeck H, Warnke PH (2001) Percutaneous treatment of chronic MRSA osteomyelitis with a novel plant-derived antiseptic. *BMC Surg* **1**: 1

Shin S, Kim JH (2005) *In vitro* inhibitory activities of essential oils from two Korean thymus species against antibiotic-resistant pathogens. *Arch Pharm Res* **28**(8): 897–901

Singh S (1999) Mechanism of action of antiinflammatory effect of fixed oil of *Ocimum basilicum Linn. Indian J Exp Biol* **37**(3): 248–52

Singh S, Majumdar DK (1999) Effect of *Ocimum sanctum* fixed oil on vascular permeability and leucocytes migration. *Indian J Exp Biol* **37**(11): 1136–8

CHAPTER 10

Can translocated bacteria reduce wound infection?

V I Nikitenko

Swab cultures from acute surgical wounds showed that *Bacillus subtilis* was the most common bacteria present. The investigators propose that the bacteria, which originate in the gastrointestinal tract, play an anti-infective role in the wound site

The composition of purulent wound exudate is being studied on an ongoing basis, but as far as we are aware there are no published papers on the identification of bacteria in the wound in the early stages of healing. A study has indicated that wound exudate may be beneficial to healing (Nikitenko, 2004). However, it has been suggested that if a wound swab indicates that bacteria are present, they should be eliminated and a sterile environment created (Kucuk et al., 2006). This study set out to determine the most common bacteria present in human wound swabs. *In vitro* and animal studies were undertaken to identify their source and determine if they are capable of exogeneous antibiotic activity.

Human study

Method

All patients undergoing surgery for open limb fractures (n=64) or osteosynthesis of closed fractures (n=73) from February 2001 to December 2006 were included. The age range was 18–86 years (mean 41). Ethical approval was given by Orenburg State Medical Academy. All patients gave informed consent. The periwound skin of all wounds was cleansed preoperatively with three antiseptics (1% povidone-iodine, 70% alcohol solution and 0.5% dioxydine) in rapid succession. At the end of each operation the wounds were swabbed with sterilised tampons. In the first three postoperative days wound exudate from between the sutures was swabbed using a microbiological loop.

Table 1. Wound microflora identified in patients during the first three postoperative days

| | Open fractures (n=64) | | Closed fractures (n=73) | |
| | At end of surgery | 1–3 days post-wounding | At end of surgery | 1–3 days post-wounding |
	No. (%)	No. (%)	No. (%)	No. (%)
No growth	52 (81)	13 (20)	58 (80)	8 (11)
Genus *Bacillus*	1 (2)	26 (41)	2 (3)	36 (49)
Staphylococcus aureus	1 (2)	2 (6)	2 (3)	3 (4)
Staphylococcus epidermidis	2 (3)	3 (5)	3 (4)	4 (6)
Staphylococcus saprophyticus	1 (2)	5 (8)	1 (2)	3 (4)
Streptococcus spp.	1 (2)	1 (2)	1 (1)	2 (3)
Enterococcus spp.	0	1 (2)	1 (1)	2 (3)
Escherichia coli	1 (2)	2 (3)	1 (1)	3 (4)
Pseudomonas aeruginosa	0	1 (2)	1 (1)	2 (3)
Klebsiella spp.	0	1 (2)	1 (1)	1 (1)
Proteus spp.	1 (2)	1 (2)	0	1 (1)
Candida	0	1 (2)	0	1 (1)
Staphylococcus aureus with genus *Bacillus*	0	1 (2)	0	1 (1)
Staphylococcus aureus with Gram-negative coccus	0	0	0	1 (11)
Staphylococcus saprophyticus or *Staphylococcus epidermidis* in association with genus *Bacillus*	1 (2)	3 (5)	2 (3)	3 (4)
Staphylococcus saprophyticus or *Staphylococcus epidermidis*	0	0	0	1 (1%)
Anaerobe*	0	2 (3)	—	—
Others	3 (5)	1 (2)	0	1 (1)
Total	64	64	73	73

15 patients with open fractures were assessed

Results

The first wound swab, taken at the end of surgery, showed there were no microorganisms in 52/64 patients with open fractures and in 58/73 patients with closed fractures. Full results are given in *Table 1*.

Open fractures

In spite of debridement of non-viable tissue and antiseptic lavage, microorganisms were identified in almost one-fifth of the patients (19%) with open fractures following wound excision. Most were monolayer cultures of *Staphylococcus epidermidis, Staphylococcus aureus, Staphylococcus saprophyticus*, Proteus and other Gram-negative *Bacillus*.

There was a marked increase in the presence of bacteria in the first three postoperative days as, in spite of the use of antiseptic bandages, wounds were sterile in only 13/64 patients (20%). This was primarily due to the onset of sporogenous Gram-positive microflora of genus *Bacillus*, which occurred in 41% of cases as a monoculture and in 6% as a polyculture.

Samples from 15 patients were cultured in anaerobic conditions, with positive results in two cases. Bacteroides were identified in one patient.

Closed fractures

Microorganisms were found in wound swabs taken at the end of surgery in only 15 of the 73 patients with closed fractures.

In the first three postoperative days the presence of bacteria increased, with only eight wounds (11%) not having any microorganisms. The most frequently identified bacterium was *Bacillus subtilis* (strains 36 and 73); in four patients it coexisted with other bacteria (*Table 1*).

Suppuration

None of the wounds of the patients in either group showed any clinical signs of suppuration in the first three postoperative days. Only a small number of bacteria was present in the wounds — no more than 10 per gram of wound exudate (Birger, 1982; Breed et al., 1974).

Genus *Bacillus* were more often identified in patients with closed fractures. Of the 73 patients, 35 were not given antibiotics during surgery and the first two postoperative days. We believe these two findings are related. The identified strains of *Bacillus subtilis* were highly sensitive to antibiotics such as penicillin, chloramphenicol, tetracycline and cephalosporin.

On the fifth postoperative day, 11 patients with open fractures and two patients with closed fractures had clinical signs of suppuration. Four patients with suppurating wounds had monocultures of *Staphylococcus aureus*,

Table 2. Relationship between the number of wounds that suppurated and the composition of the microorganisms in the wound in the first three postoperative days

	Open fractures		Closed fractures	
	No. of wounds	No. that suppurated	No. of wounds	No. that suppurated
Sterilised seedings	13	3	8	1
Staphylococcus spp.				
Enterococcus spp. etc	21	6	25	1
Genus *Bacillus*	30	2	40	0

three had Gram-negative *Enterococcus spp.* and one had *Streptococcus spp.* and *Bacteroides spp.* Bacterial combinations were found in four patients.

We analysed the relationship between the number of wounds that suppurated and the presence of the various microorganisms in the first three postoperative days. The results are given *Table 2*.

Wounds in which genus *Bacillus* was identified in the first three postoperative days of the wound-healing process were less prone to suppuration. Of the 70 patients in whom genus *Bacillus* were identified, only two (3%) had suppurating wounds. Of the 46 patients in whom other strains of bacteria were identified, seven (15%) had suppurating wounds. Similar results were recorded in the 21 patients with no bacteria in their wounds in the first three postoperative days — only four (19%) suppurated.

In vitro studies

The morphological and biochemical behaviours of the microorganisms identified in the swabs, along with their antibacterial properties, were studied using standard methodology (Birger, 1982). We also set out to determine whether any of the bacteria present showed a potential for exogenous antibiotic activity.

To identify the source of *Bacillus subtilis* in the wounds under the antiseptic bandage, we seeded bacteria from the wound swabs, periwound tissue, urine, faeces and blood of 17 patients, as well as from the treatment-room air (the latter was achieved by exposing beef-extract broth to open air for 15 minutes and then heating it to 37°C).

The results indicated that genus *Bacillus* penetrated the wound from the gastrointestinal tract: the biochemical and physiological features of the bacterial colony from the wound swabs were the same as those from blood, urine and faeces.

We then isolated strains of genus *Bacillus* from 10 wounds healing by primary intention and sent them to the Moscow Research Institute of Antibiotics, which verified that all 10 strains had antimicrobial properties. These antimicrobial properties were associated with proteinaceous structures with widely varying molecular weights.

In addition, we identified 17 strains of *Bacillus* from the wounds (Breed et al., 1974):

ı *Bacillus subtilis* — six strains
ıı *Bacillus circularis* — three strains
ı *Bacillus cereus* — two strains
ı *Bacillus pulvifaciens* — two strains
ı *Bacillus alvei* — two strains
ıı *Bacillus laterosporus* — one strain
ı *Bacillus macquariensis* — one strain.

These were grown separately in beef-extract broth, and the presence of proteolytic ferments was determined by mixing the corresponding substratum with filtered liquid (Pokrovskii, 1969).

The strains produced large numbers of proteolytic ferments that broke down albumin, protein, collagen, fat, carbohydrates and vegetable cellulose. One of the natural strains (whose number and characteristics we are unable to name as we have not yet patented it) synthesised and eliminated human fibroblast growth factors (FGF). We were unable to find any reference to such a bacterium in the literature; genetically modified strains of bacteria are used to produce fibroblast growth factors. We believe that genus *Bacillus* produces substances used in the prophylaxis and treatment of purulent inflammation.

Animal studies

Method

We undertook an animal study to identify the dosage at which administration of genus *Bacillus* would be lethal. In all, 206 mice were injected intramuscularly and subcutaneously with 10 strains of genus *Bacillus* in doses ranging from 0.5 milliard to 170 milliards in 1ml of 0.9% sodium chloride. (Both intramuscular and subcutaneous injections were used as it was thought the method of administration might affect toxicity.) The aim was to determine the dosage that would kill 50% of the animals. A strain is considered harmless if two milliards of bacteria or more fail to kill a mouse.

Intravenous (IV) and intraperitoneal infusion of the 10 strains at the above dosages did not have a toxic effect. All of the mice remained active, and did not experience any weight loss. All six mice given an IV injection of 170 milliard remained healthy. We conclude therefore that genus *Bacillus* can be considered harmless.

In a separate animal study involving 20 rabbits, we set out to determine the source of the bacteria.

To determine a safe dosage, *Bacillus subtilis* strains 534 and 538, marked with radioactive H3-leucine, were given subcutaneously at 1–5 milliards of bacteria in 1ml of 0.9% sodium chloride solution to 12 rabbits weighing 2–2.5kg each. No adverse effects occurred.

Bacillus subtilis, again marked with radioactive H3-leucine, were then administered orally into the intragastric region of eight other rabbits (four rabbits received strain 534 and four rabbits strain 538). Dosage was 1 milliard in 103 of sodium chloride. Dermal wounds 4cm long were created under inhalation anaesthesia in four of the eight rabbits (two had been given strain 534 and two strain 538). The wounds were closed and hermetically sealed with glue BF-6 to insulate them from the external environment. After a second administration of bacteria 48 hours later, the rabbits were killed with inhalation anaesthesia. Blood was collected from an ear vein shortly before this. Tissue samples were taken from the wound or skin (if the rabbits were not wounded), liver, spleen, lymph nodes from the mesentery of the small intestine, brain, lungs, stomach and large and small intestines. These samples were dissected as recommended by Ginkin (1959).

Histological analysis of the eight rabbits showed numerous radiolabels in the lymph nodes of the large and small intestines, lymphoid follice of the spleen (*Figure 1a*) and liver. Wounded rabbits had greater amounts of marked bacteria in the connective tissues of the wound area (*Figure 1b*). Some radiolabels were found in blood smears (*Figure 1c*).

In our opinion, the bacteria penetrate into blood through the desquamation areas and intercellular slots in the area of the healthy stomach and small intestine. Bacterial translocation through the mucous coat of the large intestine was not observed.

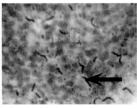
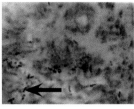
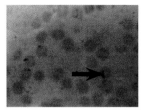

Lymphoid follicle of spleen

Connective tissue of wound

Blood smear from vein

Figure 1. Microflora in the early stages of wound healing: radiolabels of strain Bacillus subtilis 543 (see arrows). 1:1000 scale model.

Discussion

Following surgery for open or closed limb fractures most of the patients had a moderate number of *Bacillus subtilis* in their wounds in spite of the antiseptic lavage and antibiotic treatment. As far as we are aware, this is the first time this has been described in the scientific literature. As expected, the non-exuding wounds that closed up were sterile. In my opinion, bacteria living in the lumen and the periwound tissue play a key role in the healing process. This led us to conclude that the presence of *Bacillus subtilis* 534 reduces the possibility of suppuration.

The phenomenon of bacterial penetration from the gastrointestinal tract into blood and the tissues has been called 'translocation'. Most researchers regard this as a pathologic process resulting from factors such as stress, immunodeficiency and shock (Kuzin and Kostuchenok, 1981; Kane et al., 1998; Sakamoto et al., 1999; Nikitenko, 2004; Song et al., 2006). In contrast, we consider that translocation from the gastrointestinal tract through uninjured mucous coats plays an anti-infective role. As far as we are aware, these results are the first to indicate that the presence of translocated gastrointestinal microorganisms in the wound is not always harmful. Earlier work by Tenorio et al. (1976) and Levenson et al. (1983) has demonstrated the potential beneficial effect of bacteria on healing. It is possible that they could be used in the development of cheap prophylactic and anti-inflammatory drugs (Song et al., 2006).

References

Birger MO (1982) *Handbook of Methods of Microbiology and Virology* [in Russian]. Moscow Medicine

Breed RS, Murray EGD, Smith NR (eds) (1974) *Bergey's Manual of Determinative Bacteriology.* Williams and Wilkins

Ginkin LN (1959) *The usage of the radionuclides in histology. The radioactive indicators in histology.* (pp. 5–33) Leningrad, IEM AMN USSR

Kane TD, Alexander JW, Johannigman JA (1998) The detection of microbial DNA in the blood: a sensitive method for diagnosing bacteremia and/or bacterial translocation in surgical patients. *Ann Surg* **227**(1): 1–9

Kucuk C, Sozuer E, Gursoy S et al. (2006) Treatment with Met-RANTES decreases bacterial translocation in experimental colitis. *Am J Surg* **191**(1): 77–83

Kuzin MI, Kostuchenok BM (1981) *Wounds and Wound Infection* [in Russian]. Moscow

Levenson SM, KanGruber D, Gruber C et al. (1983)Wound healing accelerated by Staphylococcus aureus. *Arch Surg* **118**:310–20.

Nikitenko VI (2004) Infection prophylaxis of gunshot wounds using probiotics. *J Wound Care* **13**(9): 363–6

Pokrovskii AA (1969) *The biochemical studies in clinic* (p. 632) Moscow Medicine

Sakamoto H, Naito H, Ohta Y et al. (1999) Isolation of bacteria from cervical lymph nodes in patients wth oral cancer. *Arch Oral Biol* **44**(10): 789–93

Song D, Shi B, Xue H et al. (2006) Green fluorescent protein labeling *Escherichia coli* TG1 confirms intestinal bacterial translocation in a rat model of chemotherapy. *Curr Microbiol* **52**(1): 69–73

Tenorio A, Jindrak K, Weiner M, et al. (1976) Accelerated healing in infected wounds. *Surg Gynecol Obstet* **142**: 537–43

CHAPTER II

Efficacy of TNP on lower limb wounds: A meta-analysis

U Sadat, G Chang, A Noorani, S R Walsh, P D Hayes and K Varty

This meta-analysis of the three random controlled trials (RCTs) that have compared topical negative pressure with conventional treatment in patients with lower limb ulcers found that it significantly reduced healing times and increased the number of healed wounds.

Wound healing is a complex series of events, which are broadly classified as the inflammatory, proliferative and remodelling phases. The pathological events underlying the inflammatory stage involve haemostasis, chemotaxis and phagocytosis. The formation of granulation tissue involves angiogenesis and collagen synthesis, while healing is finally completed by neoepithelialisation.

This process is compromised in patients with arterial and/or venous insufficiency, which can prevent or delay healing, thereby increasing the risk of recurrent wound infections. Although the gold standard is to improve the arterial inflow either by angioplasty or peripheral arterial bypass surgery and to treat venous insufficiency in relevant cases, adequate localised management of the wound also facilitates the healing process.

The complexities of arterial and/or venous wounds, especially in patients with diabetes, pose a challenge for practitioners. Topical negative pressure (TNP) has emerged as an effective and novel technique that can be applied to a wide range of wounds, from clean fasciotomy wounds and skin grafts, to venous, arterial and mixed-aetiology leg ulcers (Vuerstaek et al., 2006). Patients with diabetes, who often have neuroischaemic ulcers, also benefit from the therapy (McCallon et al., 2000).

TNP is also known as negative pressure wound therapy (NPWT), sub-atmospheric pressure dressing (SPD), vacuum sealing technique (VST) and sealed surface wound suction (SSS) (Banwwell and Teot, 2003). Since the first description of TNP by Fleischmann et al. in 1993, numerous case reports and case series have reported that TNP promotes wound healing (Greer et al., 1999; Josty et al., 2001; Penn and Rayment, 2004; Scholl et al., 2004;

Ford-Dunn, 2006; Gerry et al., 2007). However, only a limited number of randomised controlled trials (RCTs) have compared it with dressings, principally dry dressings or saline-soaked dressings, and most had small sample sizes. These trials are usually heterogeneous, with each including a wide range of wounds with different aetiologies. This does not facilitate understanding of the effectiveness of TNP in specific wound types.

We present the results of a meta-analysis of RCTs involving patients with lower limb arterial and/or vascular ulcers, including diabetic foot ulcers, to assess the efficacy of TNP in the treatment of such patients. Diabetic feet were included because, despite having apparently good perfusion, there is usually an underlying vessel disease, which makes them more prone to recurrent infections and so more difficult to manage.

Method

Two independent researchers (US and PDH) carried out a systematic literature search of RCTs comparing TNP with conventional treatments in patients with lower limb wounds with underlying arterial and/or venous insufficiency. (Case reports and case-series studies were excluded.) PubMed and Embase databases from January 1993 to July 2007 were searched using the search terms 'negative wound pressure therapy', 'vacuum assisted closure' and 'wound healing'. In addition, relevant medical journals were hand searched and the references of each article retrieved were searched for missed reports. We examined the following outcome measures:

  ı   Time to healing
  ı   Number of wounds that healed with/without TNP
  ı   Infection rates in the two study groups.

Statistical analysis

StatsDirect (version 2.6.2) software was used for statistical meta-analysis. SRW abstracted the pooled data into a computerised spreadsheet for analysis.

For categorical outcomes, pooled odds ratios were calculated, using a random effects model, as described by DerSimonian and Laird (1986). For continuous outcomes, pooled effect size estimates were calculated.

Heterogeneity was tested using Cochran's Q test — a null hypothesis test in which a significant result indicates that significant heterogeneity exists. Heterogeneity can result from variable sample sizes and differences in patient demographics, the types of wounds studied and the treatments given.

The aim was to assess bias by visual inspection of funnel plots and then quantify it with the Egger test. Bias can be publication bias — that is, positive results are more likely to be published than negative, or it can result from the causes discussed in more detail above.

Meta-regression is usually performed to assess the causes of heterogeneity, but this was not possible due to the limited information provided by the RCTs identified.

All *p* values are two-sided, and the 5% level was considered significant.

Results

Three RCTs (McCallon et al., 2000; Armstrong and Lavery, 2005; Vuerstaek et al., 2006) were identified. These had a combined population of 232 patients, of whom 112 were randomised to receive Vacuum Assisted Closure (VAC, KCI, San Antonio, Texas, US) therapy and 120 to receive a control (conventional wound dressings). Details of the sample sizes, aetiologies and main results are given in *Table 1*.

Significantly more wounds healed in the VAC therapy groups, with a pooled odds ratio of 1.92 (95% confidence interval [CI]: 1.04–3.55), *p*=0.03 (*Figure 1*). There was no evidence of heterogeneity, with a Cochran Q value of 0.21, *p*=0.63.

Time to healing was also significantly shorter in the VAC therapy groups, with a pooled effect size of -1.042 (95% CI = -1.83 to -0.24), *p*=0.01 (*Figure 2*). However, heterogeneity was present, with a Cochran Q value of 10.41, *p*=0.005.

There was no difference in wound-infection rates between the two groups, with a pooled odds ratio of 1.72 (95% CI: 0.22–13.07), *p*=0.5969 (*Figure 3*). There was no evidence of heterogeneity, with a Cochran Q value of 1.76, *p*=0.18.

Due to the small number of studies, it was not possible to assess bias.

Table I. Findings of the three RCTs

Study	Aetiology	No. of patients		Healing time (days)		No. of healed wounds	
		VAC	Control	VAC	Control	VAC	Control
Vuerstaek et al. (2006)	Arterial (n=13), venous (n=13) mixed aetiology leg ulcers (n=4)	30	30	29* (CI: 25.5–32.5)	45* (CI: 36.2–53.8)	29	29
McCallon et al. (2000)	Non-infected diabetic foot ulcers	5	5	22.8 (SD: 42.8)	42.8 (SD: 32.5)	—	—
Armstrong and Lavery (2005)	Diabetic foot ulcers following partial amputation	77	85	42* (IQR: 40–56)	84* (IQR: 57–112)	43	33

*median values
CI = confidence interval; IQR = interquartile range; SD = standard deviation

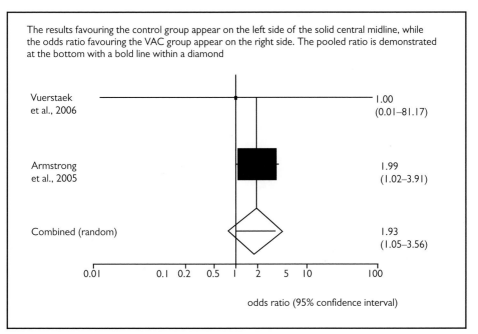

Figure 1. Forest plot showing comparing pooled odds ratio (95% confidence interval) of the healed wounds in the VAC and control group.

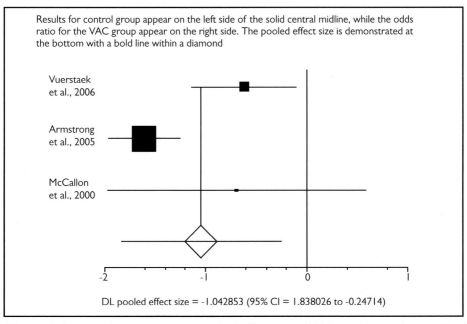

Figure 2. Forest plot comparing pooled effect size (95% confidence interval) of healing times in the VAC and control group.

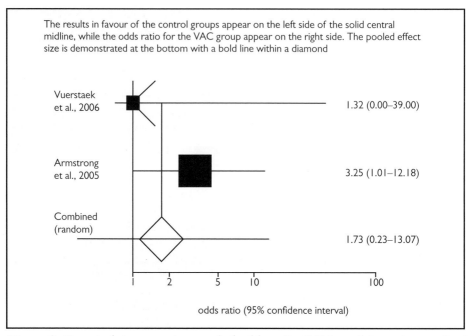

The results in favour of the control groups appear on the left side of the solid central midline, while the odds ratio for the VAC group appear on the right side. The pooled effect size is demonstrated at the bottom with a bold line within a diamond

Vuerstaek et al., 2006 — 1.32 (0.00–39.00)

Armstrong et al., 2005 — 3.25 (1.01–12.18)

Combined (random) — 1.73 (0.23–13.07)

odds ratio (95% confidence interval)

Figure 3. Forest plot comparing pooled odds ratio (95% confidence interval) of the number of infections between the VAC and control group.

Discussion and conclusion

Topical negative pressure has been used since 1993 to treat acute and chronic wounds at different sites, but gained popularity in 1997 when Argenta and Morykwas (1997) developed the VAC device to expedite healing by secondary intention. Vacuum assisted Closure involves the application of intermittent sub-atmospheric pressure of approximately 125mmHg for five to seven minutes. This negative pressure cycle is interrupted with a two-minute cycle of normal atmospheric pressure. These pressure changes increase regional blood flow by up to four times the normal rate, thereby promoting the delivery of factors that promote wound healing, such as nutrients, and maintaining an oxygen-rich environment, as well as facilitating the removal of inhibitory factors such as tissue oedema. There is also a beneficial reduction in the local bacterial count (Argenta and Morykwas, 1997; Morykwas et al., 1997; Banwell and Teot, 2003).

Topical negative pressure is therefore an effective treatment for wounds associated with arterial or venous insufficiency as it improves blood inflow and reduces tissue oedema (Argenta and Morykwas, 1997; Morykwas et al.,

1997). The mechanical stimulus resulting from the alternating pressure cycles also tends to trigger granulation tissue formation (Morykwas et al., 1997; Morykwas, 1998).In our experience, to achieve maximal benefit, the wound should be well vascularised and free of necrotic tissue before VAC is applied.

In this meta-analysis we analysed pooled data from RCTs on lower limb wounds commonly seen in vascular surgery clinics. The wounds were predominantly of diabetic aetiology. The results showed that TNP was associated with a significant reduction in healing times and an increase in the number of wounds that healed. This is despite the adverse healing responses associated with diabetic, ischaemic and mixed aetiology wounds, including impaired neutrophil chemotaxis, phagocytosis and perfusion, and the enhanced degradation of important structural proteins (Schaper and Nabuurs-Franssen, 2002).

Most RCTs involving VAC have included patients undergoing reconstructive surgery, and have found the therapy to have significant benefits (Greer et al., 1999; Josty et al., 2001; Penn and Rayment, 2004; Scholl et al., 2004; Ford-Dunn, 2006; Gerry et al., 2007).

McCallon et al. (2000) showed that VAC could halve healing times and reduce the wound size by 66% when compared with saline gauze in diabetic wounds. However, as his study included only 10 patients, statistical significance could not be reached.

A large multicentre trial by Armstrong et al. (2005) showed that more patients healed in the TNP group than in the control group, 43 (56%) versus 33 (39%), $p=0·04$. The rate of wound healing, based on time to complete closure, was faster in the TNP group than in the controls ($p=0.005$). The rate of granulation tissue formation, based on the time to cover 76–100% of the wound bed, was also faster in the TNP group ($p=0.002$). The frequency and severity of adverse events, of which the most common was wound infection, were similar in both treatment groups. However, this trial has been criticised for including surgical, as well as acute and chronic wounds. There was a high rate of infection in the TNP cohort (17% versus 6% in the control group), although the authors did not attribute this to the therapy – indeed, they failed to identify other factors that could have been responsible for this.

A recently published RCT comparing NPWT (VAC therapy) to Advanced Moist Wound Therapy (AMWT) in the treatment of diabetic foot ulcers n=342 (Blume et al 2008) found NPWT to be as safe as AMWT and superior to AMWT in terms of efficacy. The claims for equivalence in safety has been challenged by Hemkens and Waltering (2008) as they state it is unclear if for the sample size calculation safety analysis was accounted for and whether the power was sufficient. They also highlight the fact that there were more cases of infection (n = 11 vs. n = 4) and major secondary amputations observed under NPWT (n = 5 vs. n = 4) and recommend that these issues should be considered in future studies.

Vuerstack et al. (2006) have also showed that VAC resulted in a reduction in healing times.

Overall, in this meta-analysis the difference in the infection rates between the TNP and control groups was not significant, suggesting that TNP does not increase the risk of wound infection (Weed et al., 2004).

One aspect not reported consistently in the literature is the cost-effectiveness of TNP therapy. Only one RCT in our meta-analysis provided information on this (Vuerstaek et al., 2006). The total cost of treating 30 patients with TNP was $5452, compared with $38 881 for the conventional dressings group. The biggest causes of this cost difference were the higher staff costs and longer hospitalisation times associated with the slower wound healing in the control groups. Nevertheless, these figures suggest that the ability of TNP to accelerate healing does incur a moderate cost. Earlier discharge with portable TNP systems may help reduce this.

Assessment of quality of life in patients undergoing TNP has also been inconsistently reported. Since there is a strong correlation between the amount of time spent on wound care, emotional distress and patients' quality of life, there may be a quality-of-life gain for patients receiving this treatment. It may be argued that some patients may not tolerate the TNP dressing because it may worsen their pain. However, in our experience this is not common in patients with severe limb ischaemia, who are administered potent analgesics. Further studies are needed on this aspect of TNP.

Study limitations include the inclusion of studies with heterogeneous populations: Armstrong et al. (2005) recruited patients with acute and chronic wounds, while Vuerstaek et al. (2006) included patients with arterial and/or venous ulcers. Similarly, the inclusion of diabetic wounds, not all of which have an arterial component, may be responsible for the heterogeneity, and is thus a potential limitation.

Nevertheless, this meta-analysis does give a 'feel' of the efficacy of TNP in managing patients with lower limb ulcers. In addition, due to the limited information available from the published trials, it was not possible to perform a meta-regression. As the number of patients in these RCTs was small, we suggest that further evidence from multicentre controlled trials are needed to confirm these findings. This point is emphasised in a systematic review of topical negative pressure by Ubbink et al. (2008) who identified 15 publications on 13 RCTs that reported on patients with chronic wounds, diabetic wounds, pressure ulcers, skin grafts and acute wounds. This study found 15 publications on 13 RCTs evaluating its effectiveness. The authors state that these RCTs contained no aggregate evidence of more rapid complete wound healing for any type of wound. The reviewers commented on a number of flaws found in the studies and stated that together with these shortcomings (not identified here) there were little data on cost, quality of life or adverse effects, e.g. pain during foam changes. Their overall conclusions are arguably the most controversial to date: 'At present there is no worthwhile evidence to support the use of TNP in the treatment of various wounds. A far more rigorous evaluation is needed, largely in the form of RCTs. Until this has been completed, the use of TNP should not become routine or be reimbursed for local wound care.'

References

Argenta LC, Morykwas MJ (1997) Vacuum assisted closure: a new method for wound control and treatment: clinical experience. *Ann Plast Surg* **38**(6): 563–76

Armstrong DG, Lavery LA (2005) Diabetic Foot Study Consortium. Negative pressure wound therapy after partial diabetic foot amputation: a multicentre, randomised controlled trial. *Lancet* **366**: 1704–10

Banwell PE, Teot L (2003) Topical negative pressure: the evolution of a novel wound therapy. *J Wound Care* **12**(1): 28–30

Blume PA, Walters J, Payne W, Ayala J, Lantis J (2008) Comparison of negative pressure wound therapy using vacuum-assisted closure with advanced moist wound therapy in the treatment of diabetic foot ulcers: A multicenter randomized controlled trial. *Diabetes Care* **31**(4):631–6

DerSimonian R, Laird N (1986) Meta-analysis in Clinical Trials. *Controlled Clinical Trials* **7**: 177–88

Fleischmann W, Strecker W, Bombelli M, Kinzl L (1993) Vacuum sealing as treatment of soft tissue damage in open fractures. *Unfallchirurg* **96**: 488–92

Ford-Dunn S (2006) Use of vacuum assisted closure therapy in the palliation of a malignant wound. *Palliat Med* **20**(4): 447–8

Gerry R, Kwei S, Bayer L, Breuing KH (2007) Silver-impregnated vacuum-assisted closure in the treatment of recalcitrant venous stasis ulcers. *Ann Plast Surg* **59**(1): 58–62

Greer SE, Longaker MT, Margiotta M et al. (1999) The use of subatmospheric pressure dressing for the coverage of radial forearm free flap donor-site exposed tendon complications. *Ann Plast Surg* **43**(5): 551–4

Hemkins LG, Waltering A (2008) Online Letters: Comments and Responses. Response to Blume et al. (2008) Comparison of negative pressure wound therapy using vacuum-assisted closure with advanced moist wound therapy in the treatment of diabetic foot ulcers: A multicenter randomized

controlled trial. *Diabetes Care* 31:e76 2008 available at: http://care.diabetesjournals.org/cgi/
content/full/31/10/e76

Josty IC, Ramaswamy R, Laing JH (2001) Vaccum assisted closure: an alternative strategy in the management of degloving injuries of the foot. *Br J Plast Surg* **54**(4): 363–5

McCallon SK, Knight CA, Valiulus JP et al. (2000) Vacuum-assisted closure versus saline-moistened gauze in the healing of postoperative diabetic foot wounds. *Ostomy Wound Manage* **46**(8): 28–32, 34

Morykwas MJ (1998) External application of sub-atmospheric pressure and healing: mechanisms of action. *Wound Healing Soc Newsletter* **8**: 4–5

Morykwas MJ, Argenta LC, Shelton-Brown EI, McGuirt W (1997) Vacuum- assisted closure: a new method for wound control and treatment: animal studies and basic foundation. *Ann Plast Surg* **38**: 553–62

Penn E, Rayment S (2004) Management of a dehisced abdominal wound with VAC therapy. *Br J Nurs* **13**(4): 194–201

Schaper NC, Nabuurs-Franssen MH (2002) The diabetic foot: pathogenesis and clinical evaluation. *Semin Vasc Med* **2**(2): 221–8

Scholl L, Chang E, Reitz B, Chang J (2004) Sternal osteomyelitis: use of vacuum-assisted closure device as an adjunct to definitive closure with sternectomy and muscle flap reconstruction.J *Card Surg* **19**(5): 453–61

Ubbink DT, Westerbos SJ, Nelson EA, Vermeulen H (2008) A systematic review of topical negative pressure therapy for acute and chronic wounds. *Brit J Surg* **95**: 685–92

Vuerstaek DDJ, Vainas T, Wuite J et al. (2006) State-of-the-art treatment of chronic leg ulcers: a randomized controlled trial comparing vacuum-assisted closure (VAC) with modern wound dressings. *J Vasc Surg* **44**(5): 1029–37

Weed T, Ratliff C, Drake DB (2004) Quantifying bacterial bioburden during negative pressure wound therapy: does the wound VAC enhance bacterial clearance? *Ann Plast Surg* **52**: 276–9

Index

A

allograft 94
anaerobic bacteria 92
anti-biofilm agents 77
arterial
  insufficiency 128
  ulcers 124
audit
  of wounds 2
  suggestions for improvement of 13
autograft 94

B

Bacillus subtilis 115–122
bacterial profiling 91–104
basil oil 110
bioburden 93
biofilm 71–90
  infections
    treatment of 76–78
biofilm-based wound care 78
  algorithm 81
  the future 88
Burnaid cream 109

C

Cadesorb 35
cadexomer iodine 82
calendula arvensis oil 111
cell
  contraction theory 65–66
  senescence 42–43
  traction theory 66
chain reaction amplification 96
chamomile oil 108
Chromameter 23–24
Chromolaena odorata 111
chronic

venous leg ulcer 34
  wounds 34
cleansing
  of wounds 10
closed fractures 115
colonisation 92
  critical 92
complementary medicine 105
compression 7
contamination 92
contraction theories 64–67
critical
  colonisation 92
  limb ischaemia 71–90, 78–83
cultural analysis 97
Curasorb 35
Cutometer 26

D

denaturing gradient gel electrophoresis
    (DGGE) 92, 96, 97–98
Dermafex 26
DermaSpectrometer 23–24
diabetes 7, 47–62, 78
diabetic
  foot ulcers 78, 91, 124
  wound repair 56
digitiser 22
DNA
  extraction 96
  icro-array analysis system 42
Doppler 7
dressings
  for wounds 7–8
dry dressings 124
duration
  of wounds 4
Durometer 25

E

endocarditis 76
essential oils 105–114
eupolin ointment, 111
extracellular polysaccharide matrix (EPS) 93
exudate level 9

F

fibroblast culture 50
  growth factors (FGF) 119
  senescence 37–46
field marigold 111
finite element modelling 26
foot ulcer 7
fractures
  closed 117
  open 117

H

hydroxyproline 49
hyperbaric oxygen 82
Hypericum perforatum oil 111

I

incremental phase
  of healing 106
infection
  invasive 92
  local 92
  of wounds 5
invasive infection 92
ionic silver 82
ischaemia 71–90
  critical limb 78–83

K

keloid scar 22

L

lactoferrin 82
lag phase
  of healing 106

lavender oil 107–108
leg ulcers 7, 91, 93
limb ischaemia 78–83
local infection 92
lower limb wounds 123–132

M

Manchester scar scale 23
maturation phase
  of healing 106
Melaleuca 108

N

'natural' remedies 105
negative pressure wound therapy
  (NPWT) 123
nitric oxide
  role in wound healing 47–62
  synthesis 50

O

objective scar assessment 21
observer scar assessment scale 20–21
Ocimum oil 110
open fractures 115
osteomyelitis 82
oxidative stress 40

P

patient scar assessment scale 20–21
pH measurement
  for wound assessment 29–36
pliability
  of scars 24
Pneumatonometer 25
polymerase chain reaction amplification
  96
postoperative
  wound microflora 116
pressure-redistributing mattress 6
pressure
  devices 25
  ulcers 5–7, 91
    prevalence of 5–7

prevalence
  of wounds 1–16
primary dressings 9

Q

QIAmp DNA kit 96
quorum-sensing inhibitors 93

R

regional blood flow 128
repositioning schedule 6
risk assessment tool 6

S

saline-soaked dressings 124
Santiria bark oil 110
scar
  appearance of 106
  area 22
  assessment
    objective 21
    subjective 18–20
    tool 17–28
  colour 23
  dimension 22
  measurement
    non-contact methods 26
  pliability 24
  shape 22
  size 22
  thickness 22
  volume 22
sealed surface wound suction (SSS) 123
senescence 42–43
  stress induced 39–41
septicaemia 92
sequencing 99
Siam weed 111
silver-impregnated dressings 82
skin grafting 91–104
Sorbsan 35
spectrophotometric colour measurement 24
split-skin transplantation 93, 94

St John's Wort 111
stress-induced senescence 39–41
sub-atmospheric pressure dressing (SPD) 123
suction devices 26
suppuration 117–118

T

tea tree oil 108–109
telomere-dependent shortening 37–39
three-dimensional digitiser 22
thyme oil 109–110
tissue viability service 12
topical negative pressure (TNP) 123–132
torsion devices 24–25
traction theory 66
translocated bacteria 115–122
Tyco 35
type
  of wound 4

U

ulcer
  excision 93
  foot 7
  leg 7
ultrasound 22

V

vacuum sealing technique 123
Vancouver scar scale 18–19
vascular ulcers 124
venous
  insufficiency 128
  leg ulcers 93

W

Walsall score 6, 7
Waterlow score 6, 7
wound
  age 64
  audit 2
  bed
    appearance of 9

bioburden 93
care
  biofilm-based algorithm 81
cell senescence 42–43
characteristics of 6
contraction 63–70
  influences on 63–64
  theories 64–67
duration 4
healing 105–107, 123
  measurement of 29–36
  human vs. animal 64
infection 5
management 71–90
microflora 116
shape 63–64
site 64
size 30, 63–64
type 4
upregulation of 41–42
wound-healing mediators
wounds
  prevalence of 1–16

X

xenograft 94
Xylitol 82

Z

Zimmer dermatome 95